KT-225-026

Contents

Quality in the New GP Contract

Understanding, designing, planning, achieving

Andrew Spooner

*General Practitioner, Cheshire
Confederation Contract Negotiator
for the Quality and Outcome Framework
(for the GMS Contract 2002–2003)*

Foreword by

Tony Snell

RADCLIFFE MEDICAL PRESS
OXFORD • SAN FRANCISCO

Radcliffe Medical Press Ltd
18 Marcham Road
Abingdon
Oxon OX14 1AA
United Kingdom

www.radcliffe-oxford.com
The Radcliffe Medical Press electronic catalogue and online ordering facility.
Direct sales to anywhere in the world.

British Library Cataloguing in Publication Data

A catalogue record for this book is available from the British Library.

ISBN 1 85775 853 6

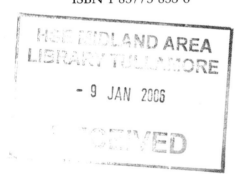
Typeset by Anne Joshua & Associates, Oxford
Printed and bound by TJ International Ltd, Padstow, Cornwall

Foreword

Quality in the New GP Contract is essential reading for GPs, practice managers and practice nurses alike. It will help them to understand the background to its structure and what to do to achieve the quality requirements.

It will also be useful for PCOs to assist them in moving to individual practice contracts. The contract will require close performance management. This book identifies the resource implications for PCOs and the personal requirements of the suitably qualified staff they will need to employ or train. The Department of Health, Strategic Health Authorities, NatPact and the Modernisation Agency would be well-advised to read the sections on implementation. There are major challenges ahead to ensure that the new contract enables the development of primary care in the context of the greatest investment in primary care since 1948 and the modernisation of the NHS.

Dr Spooner brings an academic rigour and a close personal insight into the development of the quality criteria of the new GMS contract. He has published on the primary care clinical effectiveness (PRICCE) quality improvement scheme in East Kent, the clinical model for the new contract, has been through Fellowship by Assessment of the RCGP and has assisted at the negotiations on behalf of the NHS Confederation (negotiating on behalf of the Department of Health). He has understood the objectives of the 'union' (the GPC of the BMA) and the employers, and has used the research evidence and knowledge of everyday practice to show how the Quality and Outcomes Framework was developed.

Dr Spooner comprehensively reviews the issues around the relationship of clinical governance to the quality contract. The Quality and Outcomes Framework maps across to the current seven pillars of the Commission for Health Improvement. It will provide a more acceptable set of clinical indicators for the new Commission for Healthcare Audit and Inspection to measure PCOs' improvement.

Part 3 of the book takes us through the range of practices and how each of them will need to change to meet the significant challenge set by the contract in their own context. He suggests the steps practices will need to consider and implement. This is laid out in a sensible business and project planning way for each of the main change areas, such as IM&T, training, practice management, skill mix, chronic disease management, medicines management and finance.

The accurate clinical data that practices will produce will provide PCOs with the information to reveal gaps in commissioning (e.g. echocardiography) and will enable research. It will provide public health departments with a mass of information that should aid the reduction of inequalities in access, and quality of services, as well as targeting primary and secondary prevention.

I commend this book as a significant tool in the implementation of the new GMS contract and the modernisation of primary care.

Dr Tony Snell MBChB DRCOG MRCGP
Medical Director
Birmingham and the Black Country Strategic Health Authority
Co-Vice Chair
NHS Confederation GMS Negotiating Team (Quality Lead)
October 2003

Preface

A new GP contract has been agreed between government and doctors'
representatives.[1] It contains a Quality and Outcomes Framework which
lists quality standards to foster and reward a particular type of practice.
There are rules about the minimum requirements to work for the state, a
series of payments dependent on patient numbers and a series of voluntary
additional payments for performing quality to a specified standard. The
contract is between the PCO and the GP practice. It replaces a contract
with individual doctors where some specified tasks were paid for and some
organisational requirements funded as reimbursements. Both contracts are
for the provision of a complex service and much more than a contract of
employment with individuals. A contract of this type is only possible
because individual practices are in place and capable of independent action
and improvement.

Practices and managers will find it helpful to understand the environment
that caused it to be written and the evidence used to construct the contract.
The management organisations for primary care have recently changed.[2] They
have a requirement to involve professionals in management and quality
improvement.[3] Managers and clinicians seek to improve healthcare from
different perspectives and with different resources. The contract provides a
mechanism to assist GP practices and PCOs in that task. There is a lot of
published work on change management in medicine. This contract has drawn
on the principles used in successful change management to create a new
entity. It aims to exploit the features of British general practice where senior
generalist doctors provide comprehensive care for most illnesses, are personally available to patients and manage a small business to provide that
service.

The contract aims to produce better outcomes and improved mortality and
morbidity for patients. New patient agendas of improving access to care,
involvement in service planning and autonomy in decision making for
individual patients are included. It is also intended to start the process of
restoring the self-belief and morale of practitioners.

This book aims to document the reasons for the creation of the contract, the
change management methods used before and the features of general practice
it seeks to exploit. It then shows how they can be used to create quality
markers in other settings. Those principles are used to describe how the
specific arrangements for the new contract were derived.

This is followed by a description of the organisation that is intended to
develop and some useful methodologies to make those changes. The additional tasks that practices need to perform to succeed with the new contract
are described. There are examples of successful methods. It draws out the
implications for the practice and how GP partners and staff relate to each other

in a developed practice. Methods to ensure that quality is happening and steer the practice are described. There are examples of the changes that need to be made to the partners' working arrangements to manage a large and complex organisation. It is success with delegation and management that will allow practices to achieve high-quality healthcare with a manageable workload and improved morale for all who work there.

The tools required to understand the current capability of a practice and meet all the criteria of the contract are described. A method of transferring this to a business plan and practice professional development plan follows. The text does not give detailed practice procedures and clinical protocols because these should be created locally and change rapidly. The process of creating them is itself beneficial.

Achieving quality in the new contract with controlled expenses will result in significant rises in incomes. Understanding how and why the contract was written and using the tools to succeed will help a practice to be among the high earners and leave it well placed for future change.

The practice can use its control of resources and workload with reduced external control. That will allow it to organise itself efficiently and achieve challenging quality markers, something of which it can be justifiably proud.

The book will be of interest to those wishing to understand the contract or design another one. It will also help GPs, practice staff and PCO managers to understand the advantages of using the GP practice as an organisational structure and to unleash the potential to radically alter the care received by patients. The contract aims to exploit that inherent potential of general practice. Explaining why it was done and how the task can be accomplished will help that.

Andrew Spooner
October 2003

About the author

Andrew Spooner is currently a full-time GP in Crewe, Cheshire. His practice has undergone the change from reactive disease management to systematic care of illness. It seemed clear to him that the best UK general practice could be cost effective, extremely high quality and deliver care to whole populations whilst being a rewarding place to work. This led him to a search for an accepted method of quality improvement and management development for practices.

Andrew has spent time investigating change management in many spheres and relating ideas to the real situation of a challenging practice environment and he has undertaken and published an evaluation of the PRICCE scheme in East Kent. He also participated in Fellowship by Assessment and helped with the development of Membership by Assessment of the RCGP.

In June 2002 he was appointed as an NHS Confederation negotiator for the new GMS contract quality group. This group negotiated the Quality and Outcomes Framework of the new contract.

Part 1

Why the contract was created

Chapter 1

Why is there a need for a new contract?

General practice is a wonderful career

General practice used to be highly regarded as a career. It had good recruitment of general practitioners (GPs) with large numbers of high-quality applicants for most vacancies. The number of GPs increased each year. The job itself was fun and interesting to do, with increasing quality clinical care and continuity provided to patients. The patients usually appreciated the service, respected the GP and valued contact with the practice. Income was satisfactory and access to appointments was typically within a few days. It wasn't that long ago and many involved with general practice reading this book will remember the good times. The basis of general practice is still there but current evidence suggests that GPs have low morale and numbers are increasing very slowly. There is a need to rediscover a satisfying career that meets the needs of patients, provides good clinical care and well-remunerated enjoyable employment. General practice was and can be a satisfying place to work that brings real health gain to patients.

Times have changed. The focus has moved from the individual GP providing a service to a team. Treatments are now available for chronic illnesses that will treat symptoms and extend the length of life. There is evidence that their use will reduce premature death.[4] It has been calculated that 80% of the interventions in cardiology that will extend life should be delivered in primary care.[5] Patients want to be involved in their treatment and service and will no longer accept someone else deciding for them. The way lives are lived, the diet people eat, stress in their lives, whether they smoke or not all profoundly affect their health.[6]

This new agenda should be good for general practice. Most patient contacts are in general practice and therefore it has a major role in these areas. If beneficial change is to occur there is a need for more availability, spreading the load across a team, comprehensive treatment of chronic illness and effective lifestyle advice.[7] This has been happening in practices for years and GPs can take pride in leading that process. The analysis of the existing problem seeks to understand what is causing the decline in morale and to maximise the improvement in care with the available resources.

What is being requested?

In order to implement this agenda there was a need to reduce the variability of the existing service[8] and to bring all practices up to the level of the best. The new tasks in chronic disease management and patient empowerment need to be achieved. The attractiveness of general practice as a career needs to improve to address the morale and recruitment problems.[9,10] The finance to support greater numbers of primary care professionals in general practice must be provided.

GPs have requested an increase in income and a reduction of workload.[11] The nature of a small business forces GPs to decide between maximising income and reducing workload because the partners' income is the remainder after expenses. If more people are employed or investment improves efficiency, the work reduces but so does income. There is thus a need for increased practice resources and a steady and increasing supply of staff of all types.

The reasons for the feelings of disengagement and burnout need to be explored.[12] Exit surveys of people leaving general practice and the public services show that autonomy over the treatment methods used and the organisation of the working environment are important in individuals' decision to leave.[13] The environment and management system will need to change to accommodate this.

The practice workforce now has more part-time workers who require different hours to fit with other commitments.[14] For some it will be family commitments or childcare. For others it will be a portfolio career within medicine. Learning about a specialist area in clinical medicine within the practice or other areas outside it requires a reduced time commitment in the practice. Fewer GPs are taking on partnerships and the investment in the practice infrastructure.[9,10] At different stages of an individual's career all these factors may be relevant so the employment arrangements need to be flexible.

Responsibility for health has been devolved to England, Scotland, Wales and Northern Ireland. Each government has different views but general practice has one national contract across the four countries. The contract was negotiated by a collective representative, the NHS Confederation. Many of the documents and structures familiar to English readers are different in the other countries. For example, the National Institute for Clinical Excellence (NICE) and National Service Frameworks (NSFs) are replaced by the Scottish Intercollegiate Guideline Network (SIGN) and National Priorities, which are broadly similar but not identical. The detail of access targets in England and Scotland, for example, is different. The management organisation for general practice in each country is different in name and function. The generic term 'primary care organisation' (PCO) has been used throughout this book.

The negotiating priorities were not framed by any one national government and also include the aspirations of managers who work in the health service. The contract had to be agreed with the governments of all four countries. The four UK governments wanted to measure what was being achieved in chronic disease management and prove that high levels were being maintained. There was also a desire to measure and facilitate patient access within a specified time. This was to be achieved in an efficient manner with appropriate delegation of the clinical and managerial tasks. This would allow good use to be made of GPs' and other staff time to produce an efficient service. This requires targeting of resources and some control. There was also a request for local feedback and change in response to patients' views.

It is policy for more patients to be treated in primary care.[7] This led to a desire to increase the proportion and complexity of care carried out in the community.

There is a wish to ensure that specific defined clinical tasks are achieved within a reasonable time and that medical practice is updated as it becomes clear that old methods of practice are damaging or inappropriate.

Chapter 2

Previous attempts at improving primary care

General practitioners hold individual contracts with the NHS. They are organised as practices which employ staff and own facilities, function as partnerships and are independent businesses. The NHS employs managers in each local area and requires them to meet its objectives. The detail of the contract with the NHS, the relationship with the local management structure and the requirements the NHS puts on managers have been the dominant influences on changes and improvement in general practice.

GP contracts

The 1966 contract and its terms and conditions of service were effective in improving general practice. It provided a framework for sustained investment in GPs, practice staff, premises and supporting infrastructure. Progress was variable but GPs accepted the quality markers of the day. Contraception, maternity care, vaccinations and smears were performed in practices and these services were offered to most patients. Once these baseline values had been attained there was considerable autonomy for practices to utilise their own time or staff time to develop new areas of interest. There was professional support and every year the number of whole-time equivalent GPs increased.[10] Specific vocational training requirements were introduced and recruitment was adequate.

Later, managers were employed within practices and new tasks were taken on. Some practices became progressively more organised and developed disease indexes and the systematic care of chronic illnesses. As computers became more widespread, these records and registers became computerised and practices used this new ability to audit their own work.

1966 contract

- Quality markers introduced to most practices
- Diverse development agenda
- Recruitment adequate
- Variable standard of care and investment
- Couldn't be cash limited
- Costly through local duplication and falling list sizes

Unfortunately the cost of this system was high because every facility had to be provided in every practice. Some practices invested heavily and expensively yet there was no ability to create a uniform service. In some practices standards are not as high and facilities were not provided. This was addressed by a more managerial approach, the cash limiting of the additional money for reimbursement of staff and premises. Specific quality schemes were introduced for prescribing and some markers of quality. In 1990 these changes could not be agreed with the profession and a new contract was imposed as a change to the terms and conditions of service.

Some of the quality markers were accepted as a good thing and the uptake of vaccinations and smears improved after the introduction of the contract. The targets had no provision for patient choice and practice pay was directly linked to specific levels of achievement. Many did not like targets used in this way. It also increased motivation around specific levels but left minimal or no incentive above the maximum level or well below each individual level. Other areas, including elderly person checks and the health promotion scheme, were not accepted, possibly because GPs could not be convinced that they would improve the care of patients. Over time those schemes were refined, changed or ignored.

The proportion of income from capitation was increased. This favoured large list sizes and encouraged GPs to delegate work to others within the practice. The supervising managers gained the ability to decide where funding was required and new cash limits were introduced on the spending on infrastructure.

1990 contract

- Updated quality markers
- Managerial approach to reduce variability
- Rewards to favour large list sizes
- Cash limiting of expenses

Fundholding was also introduced in 1990. Here fixed budgets were set for the cost elements of the GP practice (GP staff, prescribing and referrals). Some felt this was successful as a mechanism to limit prescribing and referral cost and to provide finance to develop practices. Increased practice management occurred under the strategic leadership of the GPs. In some practices there was major development of facilities but ultimately, because the task set was financial, it could not be justified against the charge of putting patient care below income considerations. The funding was based on historical costs and consequently varied widely, even in similar areas. This could not be justified yet there were too many vested interests to change the funding formula.

Consequently the innovative change of the 1990 contract did not reduce the variability of service delivery either for the care of GP patients or for those referred. The low morale of GPs was discussed and GP trainee numbers fell but surveys of morale showed a reduction after 1990 that recovered by the mid-1990s.[15]

In recent years the movement to evidence-based medicine has been harnessed to create NICE and SIGN. This allowed the creation of single solutions to problems and the promulgation of process-based methods of reducing variation between practices. This rests on the assumption that there is one method of best practice in any individual situation. NICE does not produce implementation methods but the amount and sophistication of local management for primary care have been increased, so enhancing control over prescribing, computing, practice development and investment and clinical pathways.

Computer software was developed to encourage specific treatment paths to be followed. Specific government initiatives like Prodigy remain unused in practices.[16] Morale and job satisfaction have reduced to such an extent that retention of existing GPs is a problem.[14] Surveys now show that job satisfaction is the factor responsible for this decline, expressed as an intention to leave. Partnerships are no longer the only route to a career in practice for a doctor. The number of non-partners and locums has increased which reduces the number available to invest in infrastructure, premises and practice management.

2002 problems and changes

- Poor morale and recruitment
- Variable clinical care
- Reducing proportion of GP partners

One attempt at providing a solution to all these problems was the practice-based contract of Personal Medical Services (PMS). Here the GP practice receives a global sum of money in return for meeting specific objectives agreed with the local PCO. This provided evidence that the profession was willing to look at different markers of quality and could achieve disease management across a practice. Some of these pilots involved professionals other than GPs in the management of the organisation. This has led to a desire to allow contracts with different staff within the primary care team and removal of the requirement to contract only with GPs. Unfortunately, while there is evidence that PMS practices have more resources at their disposal, there is little evidence that they are performing better than other practices or that recruitment is better.[17]

Managerial structures

Along with changes in the GP contract have come parallel changes in the management structures. The 1966 contract was not managed; it was administered by family practitioner committees (FPC). The practitioners had guaranteed access to funds for specified developments such as premises and staff and the practice had the right to use that to obtain resources provided they met some requirements. For example, the limit on premises spending was a maximum area of building in square feet that could be reimbursed and the limit on staff was two per GP principal. Funding was not cash limited. The FPC retained an overview of the local situation and could encourage but could not force practices to develop. Some practices wanted to expand beyond these limits while others did not develop at all. The resources and management structure was separate from the hospital service.

In 1990 the FPCs were replaced by family health service authorities (FHSA) which had a managerial role in deciding where money should be spent and dividing up a cash limited sum between practices for staff and premises.[18] Their entire remit was primary care and their funding could only be spent in general practice (medical, dental and optometry). They were part of health authorities which had responsibility for the hospital service as well. Most of their spending was in hospitals and community services. At this time fundholding (practice-based purchasing of a limited number of services) was introduced and whilst the management of fundholding fell to health authorities, FHSAs had a role in helping practices to develop and expand managerial capacity to run the fund. Health authorities worked more closely with FHSAs than they had with FPCs. As the capacity of primary care expanded it became more important to the local health economy. Consequently more managerial pressure was exerted on practices to deliver services in specified ways.

In 1997 there was a change of direction.[19] Individual practice purchasing was ended in England, Wales and Scotland and replaced by area purchasing within new PCOs. These organisations had clinicians at a senior and representative level. PCOs were allocated a unified budget for primary and secondary care and asked to invest in primary care, in place of primary care-based purchasing. They retained responsibility for managing GP practices and acquired a new responsibility for quality. Previously managers had some responsibility for quality but now it became a more significant part of their role. This was to be achieved by clinical governance (defined as improvement in medical care by avoiding risk, investigating and learning from mistakes and disseminating good practice). This replaced the previous system of professional self-regulation. A new organisation, the National Institute for Clinical Excellence (NICE), was established to use evidence to decide on best practice in any area.

Clinical governance and the methods to be used were further refined in England to a system where NICE would produce guidance and NSFs would decide priorities and investment plans for specific areas of practice (e.g. cardiovascular disease or care of the elderly).[20] These would be decided centrally as a series of guidelines and protocols that would be implemented locally through clinical governance arrangements in the PCO. The level of achievement would be checked by inspections from the Commission for Health Improvement (CHI). This became a process-dominated system as managers did not all have clinical skills and could not challenge clinicians directly. They acquired national or local guidelines from other clinicians, usually experts in the field concerned, and enforced or encouraged their adoption. Practices were encouraged to develop themselves and PCOs became organisers of education.

Devolution of the NHS to the four UK governing bodies occurred in 1999. Subsequently the requirements and responsibilities of PCOs started to diverge and different plans and policies were developed in each country. After this date documents only refer to one country although the aims of the health services have remained similar.

The NHS Plan set out the priorities for investment in primary care and the rest of the health service. It described the number of new staff and requested reduced demarcation between job roles and a flexible workforce. The Modernisation Agency was created to help clinicians redesign services. Patient views were to be more important in service design and used to shape services at all levels. This was particularly important for PCOs as the commissioner of services. The responsibilities of the English PCOs were defined in the following year.[3] This devolved power for commissioning to primary care trusts (PCTs) for most primary and secondary care. Working practices were to change to give more power to frontline staff. Patients were to be involved as the arbiters of service provision. GP specialists were to be developed to allow a greater proportion of care to be delivered outside hospital. Inspections by CHI and performance management to targets set by government were continued.

PCOs have responsibility for implementing government targets which differ slightly in the four UK countries. PCOs have power as commissioners of care and resources to spend. They have a direct management responsibility for general practices but few direct controls. Clinicians are to be involved in change and encouraged to develop but encouraging specific processes to be used is more difficult when power is devolved to clinicians. PCOs are inspected on a regular basis to review their performance. CHI has now developed requirements for clinical governance that PCOs are required to meet.

The problems to be solved by managers are how to persuade the organisations they contract with, in this case general practices, to focus their resources on the PCO's clinical governance priorities. A method is required to achieve development and provide a quality assured service that is accessible to patients. The principal influence over GP practices is the national GP contract. The negotiation of a new GMS contract provides an opportunity to align PCO and GP practice priorities with a successful change management method.

Chapter 3

The existing general practice structure

The current structure of UK general practice is multiple small units. There is supporting structure (existing premises and employed staff) which allows the doctors to own and strategically manage a practice. Investment is controlled by the doctors but payments and reimbursements encourage specific developments for premises, computers and staff. The units are autonomous and there is no direct observation of what happens in a practice. There is help from PCOs for investment projects and management support.

This structure allows very good and very poor practice in each individual area. At its best clinical care is up to date and clinical knowledge is used to rapidly change practice structures and investment to focus development on the creation of open accessible services for patients. If there is progress in any clinical area it can be assimilated and patient care changed rapidly. Practices can change computer data entry methods, staff and premises to accomplish the new way of delivering patient care. If problems arise they are brought rapidly to the attention of the senior managers in the system (the GPs) and solutions developed locally and cheaply. This can only happen because a senior person in the organisation is personally overseeing the throughput of the organisation. There is the ability to manage much illness within the organisation but to use external services when needed in a targeted way. The advice of many different external services can be integrated and decisions made between the potentially conflicting advice.

At its worst all the same attributes can be used to produce a poor management environment. Clinical care can be poor or outdated. Staff can be exploited and very little produced with large inputs of resources. There is no method to force engagement. Investment can be poorly targeted or based on incorrect aims that do not improve care for patients. The ability to refer can be over- or underused. Internal disputes between the doctors can damage the business and reduce the ability to develop or use resources through inappropriate arguments.

Those charged with managing the system find they have little ability to monitor the most basic of information. They are not confident of their ability to influence practices.[21] The information that is produced by the old GMS contract does not help with the complex issues involved. The job of the GP is complicated and requires judgement. It is difficult to be sure externally if the correct clinical decisions have been taken. Investment in practice premises, staff and IT is variable and not related to deprivation.[8] Investment varies within and between PCOs. The same variation is seen in the achievement of universal chronic disease management. Complaints and safety issues are monitored but provide random pieces of information. The existing disciplinary arrangements are hard to use because targeting of problems is difficult.

Review has shown that practices do not use the priorities of the service to create their business plans and feel able to plan independently of the service.[22] GPs do not develop coherent plans to meet specified long-term goals like the control of chronic disease. The information they collect is variable and some is redundant. They are good at managing themselves and responding to local opportunities using the resources of the NHS but not necessarily at using local data to plan and focus on NHS priorities.

Those who purchase and administer healthcare cannot allow variable practice so a method is required to raise standards and stop poor practice. There are therefore two possible ways of proceeding. They could specify exactly what will be done as a series of process measures for both management structure and clinical actions. Alternatively a system could be developed to change the environment and encourage improvement across general practice whilst leaving control of the organisation where it is. In either case the aim is to increase the number of average or poor practices that perform as well as the best.

Table 3.1 The advantages and disadvantages of GP organisational structure.

	Best	Worst	What is observed
Clinical freedom	Can innovate and control the organisational environment to facilitate clinical work	Can do the minimum and perform poorly. Can block development GPs don't like	Variability and occasional poor practice. Good practice obvious to patients and invisible to the system
Organisational freedom	Innovation and good staff relations, leadership	Abuse of staff, bullying in poorly paid positions doing most of the work	Practices are less bureaucratic than other NHS employers and able to recruit from elsewhere. Some evidence of very poor practice and employment disputes
Business focus	Focused on the patient Focused on PCO agenda potential conflict	Focused on internal argument or time off, minimal service provision. Focused on neither patient nor PCO	High patient satisfaction rating with occasional problems
Size of organisation Control of investment	Focuses on paid task and reduction of additional spending, keeping the organisation lean and efficient	Minimal provision and investment, poor quality or absent facilities. Some don't meet statutory minimum requirement	No data on outputs therefore no method of assessing
Investment targeting	Integration of clinical priorities and investment to overcome blocks to progress	Poor-quality high-cost investment decisions on a whim for unnecessary cost	No data on outputs therefore no method of assessing
Position in local community	Can pick up the feeling of the community and patients and provide tailor-made locally appropriate solution	Can ignore local and national feeling and create a provider-driven service	High patient satisfaction rating with occasional problems
Breadth of clinical ability	Can tackle many issues at one consultation and integrate the diagnosis and care of many symptoms to produce a single patient-centred treatment plan	Can retreat into small scope of care and refer all other cases elsewhere	High patient satisfaction rating with occasional problems
Adaptability	Ability to see an agenda, change frequently to train for and implement clinical and organisational change	Inflexible and refuse to produce up-to-date clinical care	Most adapt well and chronic disease management figures slowly improving
Small organisation in a wider structure	Can share collective resource above practice level for specific tasks: • Financial risk sharing • Clinical support and education • Professional associations • Postgraduate structures • Workforce training (undergraduate and postgraduate)	Ignores wider structure, isolated	Managers feel unable to influence in specific directions when the government has priorities
Direct observation	Participates voluntarily in assessment schemes	Fraud and crime can continue without observation or action	Well-publicised failures, no data on the successes

Chapter 4

Methods used to produce change

What has to be achieved to produce quality

Medicine constantly changes. New information constantly becomes available. Some established teaching methods become out of date and need to be changed. This applies to clinical methods and practice organisation. New treatments are introduced slowly but when it becomes apparent that a substantive body of evidence exists that a new treatment is better than another, it is the responsibility of the health services to make treatments available to all and this should not depend on the local circumstances or the individual clinician.[19,20]

Even before contact with medical services, the lifestyle of the patient profoundly affects the prevalence of disease.[6] For this reason advice on lifestyle that leads to change is important. General practice makes 80% of all patient contacts so it is in a good position to offer advice and help for patients wishing to change.[8]

As primary care sees most patients and the patients have to be identified before any intervention can take place, it is necessary to find patients with particular illnesses. The large percentage of patients seen routinely and the single point of contact allow population screening for illness. Once identified, records and registers can be created and optimal patient management introduced for all patients.

There is a need for a method that allows advances in medicine to be reliably implemented across general practice, particularly for chronic disease management. General practice has a role in diagnosis, treatment, referral and support of patients. Chronic disease management is a part of medicine and by no means the only important task of general practice. Other areas are important but more difficult to measure. Best practice is required for all areas of medicine. Whilst figures exist in a few disease areas the principle of using evidence to find better ways to deliver care and implement best practice widely applies to all of medicine.

In order to produce change there has to be the capacity and ability to perform existing and new work. This requires development of individuals and their organisation, the practice. The creation of knowledge and skills will produce benefit in the areas measured for quality. Development will also bring the ability to produce improvement in new or unmeasured areas.

It is government policy that patients should be involved in decisions about how services are provided. Similarly, access to care is required and the four governments have specified what should happen in each country. Both are quality issues and the change implementation mechanism should include these areas.

The method of implementation should be acceptable to those charged with introduction of the measure and maintain or improve their morale and job satisfaction. This is the agenda of clinical governance but there are many ways to make it happen and the most obvious or intuitive are not always the most effective.

In order to address this situation it is necessary to look at the individual methods and schemes used to produce change to understand their effects and create a new management method to produce consistently high-quality care for patients.

Use of guidelines

Medicine has always looked to research to find the best method for any particular set of circumstances. Such is the volume of research that individual practitioners cannot keep up with the new evidence in any area of medicine. Consequently experts collate the evidence and create statements of current best practice. These are then made available to the wider profession. This is the implementation phase, which is usually written documents sent to individuals or decision support aids embedded in information technology.

In order to change practice the written document has to be accepted and used by the target audience of professionals. There are different strengths of advice. At the lowest level there is education of the recipient. They are free to accept or reject the advice. Then there is guidance where it is expected that the advice will be followed. A guideline is more detailed and stronger and finally a protocol is expected to be followed.

Hierarchy of advice to practitioners

- Education
- Guidance
- Guideline
- Protocol

Unfortunately detailed review of the effects of using guidelines and protocols alone as the primary driver for change has confirmed their inability to influence clinicians.[23] Disseminating guidelines through continuing medical education alone is not thought to result in change and nor is mailing educational materials on prescribing. Decision support is partially effective and improves the apparent care of specific diagnoses but the net effect is small as the diagnosis changes and the treatment stays the same. If change has a local champion it sometimes occurs but the effect is variable. The reasons why interventions work in one setting and not in another are not clear.

It is thought that guidelines as part of schemes can be effective. The context of the local scheme and how it works with the characteristics of the local area, the beliefs and attitudes of the clinicians and whether local leaders support the change are important for implementation. These issues are discussed in detail later for a single example scheme.[24]

Effect on changing care
- Guidelines as a primary tool are largely ineffective
- Decision support software is minimally effective
- Creating or enabling local leaders sometimes works
- Education alone does not produce change
- Schemes involving them all sometimes work

The lack of effect from guidelines seems counterintuitive. It seems appropriate to create a solution and give it to others to implement. However, the detail of guideline writing and dissemination creates a number of problems.

A guideline originates with an idea: a problem that has to be solved, how to treat a particular clinical situation or an attempt to encourage the use of a particular treatment. This is followed by the recruitment of a professional or a group to write the guideline. Experts are usually chosen but, by definition, anyone with special knowledge must be different from the target group of clinicians. The experts specify a series of actions to be followed – the guideline. If this is already happening it will be accepted but no change will occur because it was previously implemented. If it isn't current practice, it has to be disseminated. The recipients of the guideline are busy people and they receive a lot of information. A proportion of guidelines will fail because they are not read or understood and the specific change requested is not noticed.

Even if they are read in detail, the clinician may not agree with the guideline and reject the advice.[25] This could be because the clinician does not agree with the aim of the guideline or because there is something in the method requested that they do not agree with. Externally the system cannot discern the reason for the lack of implementation. A few clinicians will produce objections but most will just quietly ignore the guideline.

If an individual agrees with the principle of the guideline it may still not be implemented, possibly because of clinical or organisational factors that could be quite specific to the local environment. It may be too difficult because a measurement is not available or takes too much time to do in a surgery environment. It may be due to lack of resources in staff, finances or equipment. The guideline often does not come with resources to use for implementation. Even if resources are made available they may be used for other purposes. In individual cases it may not be the correct solution for the patient. All of this leads to partial implementation. It is not clear to anyone auditing the system which of these reasons is responsible for non-implementation. When research is done these factors are listed as blocks to implementation.[26]

As guidelines and techniques become more sophisticated these reasons are steadily stripped out. As a computer is used to suggest solutions and guide clinical management down pathways, options disappear. If the problem was lack of access to the guideline then implementation will improve without penalty. If the problem is that the clinician feels the guideline is wrong, he or she will find ways to avoid the guideline, for example by changing the diagnosis to allow them to follow a different pathway.[23] If resources are provided this will help. If the problem was organisational it can be solved but if the professional doesn't agree with the guideline, they will resist it.[27] Eventually a point is reached where they are forced to do something they do not agree with and feel is professionally wrong.

At this point the guideline or protocol becomes damaging to the professional. They are forced to do what they believe is incorrect or they give up and leave. Most of the time it will not go this far. The protocol or guideline is not implemented and the clinicians become unhappy.

This is inevitable if new ways of working are to be introduced for all by this method. Because it is the guideline that is being enforced, not the desired outcome directly, the focus of the clinicians' discomfort becomes the guideline. There is no consideration by the clinician of the improvement in care requested, only of the process issues of the guideline. It is not appropriate to continue with outdated practice but the price is high if this implementation method is used.

So far the discussion has been about implementation of clinical care by guideline but the same principles apply to using guidelines to implement specific staff structures or other management policies. The development agenda of clinical governance is being introduced in this way.[8] The number of new initiatives leads to the additional problem of overload due to the number of guidelines and protocols that have to be used. Even in the small area of prescribing, the generalist role requires the GP to implement a large number of initiatives, some of which are measured, leading to a feeling of domination and control.[13]

Implementing change by guideline and protocol introduces many opportunities to upset the individual professional and increases the risk of harm. The literature on guideline implementation is large but there is relatively little about the effect that introducing guidelines has on the individuals who are expected to implement them. There is a small body of evidence to show that as control is increased, either to introduce guidelines or for other purposes, physicians become steadily more disengaged from the management process and burnout increases.[28] This combination of burnout and disengagement was found in Scottish GPs.[12] The Audit Commission found that the reduction in autonomy for individuals inherent in this process is in part responsible for the decision to leave public service.[13]

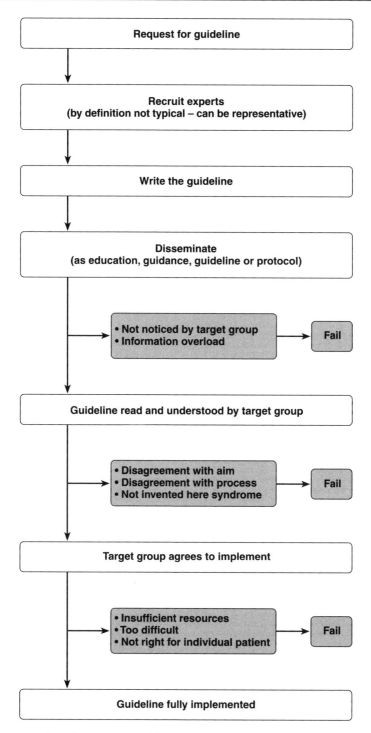

Figure 4.1 Protocol implementation problems.

Learning from management outside medicine

The difficulties of achieving uniform and repeated change in an organisation to stay up to date also exist in general management outside medicine. Business has considered many solutions and control from above is not usually considered the most effective.

Total quality management (TQM) took these principles and produced a specific method to continuously improve quality.[29] The business clearly states its aim and all levels in the organisation are encouraged to produce ideas to allow improvement. Often the most effective ideas come from those who do the job. Each idea is formulated into a plan to improve a process. This is then introduced in one area of a business and observed and audited to see if it has been successful. In manufacturing industry the change in efficiency can be small. Statistical methods are used to decide from the audit whether beneficial change has occurred. The business repeats the 'plan, do, study, act' (PDSA) cycle to test different methods of improvement. The improvement cycles are run by managers who collect and control the audit data and set the aim of the business. The worker produces the ideas but does not control their own job. When new methods or processes are found to be efficient the principles are described and introduced widely with further local consultation but without local control.

In large, centrally run organisations local managers and workers have to accept the solutions they are given. Something local may be causing inefficiency in the plant but only central rules can be followed. This sort of problem is common in large organisations and is affected by the way the organisation is managed.[30,31] The business specifies rules and ways of working that are thought to be efficient. They cannot be adapted and only single solutions to problems can be followed whether they improve efficiency or not. Local managers then have to spend time finding ways to get round the rules to be able to run the service rather than using locally appropriate, efficient solutions.

Box 4.1 Introducing single methods everywhere will create local inefficiencies

Example: nurse triage is always a good idea

There is an assumption that patients wish to see GPs for problems that do not require their skills and that many requests for GP appointments, particularly urgent ones, can be triaged to another service, usually nurse led. This was required to be introduced in order to release additional funding which could only be used for this purpose. However, a long-term policy of patient education and not prescribing antibiotics had reduced the inappropriate demand for emergency appointments. A survey of emergency patients revealed that the vast majority were being seen appropriately.

A triage service was set up. Patients requesting appointments were rung back and the emergency appointments were moved to the afternoon. Most patients were given appointments the same day. The receptionists were unhappy at having to create lists of patients and the additional work in handling phone calls, whilst nurses felt they were acting as receptionists and merely making appointments. Demand for appointments was not significantly affected. Patients waited longer and had additional inconvenience in obtaining an appointment. Cost increased, efficiency decreased and staff satisfaction reduced.

In many practices nurse triage will be a good idea but one size doesn't fit all. A less specific approach could have used the nurse time in more efficient and satisfying ways to release doctor time and improve care.

The experience of the workers in any organisation gives opportunities to use their ability and the detailed local knowledge of the problems to improve efficiency.[30] In order to do this the worker takes on a management role. The business clearly states what it wants to achieve and motivates the worker to improve his or her own job. The rules and values of the company are stated to support the worker and to set limits on the amount of change open to the worker. Advice and guidance are given but the decisions remain in the hands of the workers themselves. Some form of monitoring system is required to check the system is working and that the individual can cope with the responsibility. The examples given are diverse and include telephone repairmen and surgeons organising the use of operating theatres. As the reasons why systems don't work well are often local, large improvements in productivity are produced by small changes at low cost. The worker has more control and they feel better. This is not the same as TQM although the PDSA cycles are similar. Every individual or subunit analyses and makes changes rather than one unit experimenting and others adopting the best method. Support and common solutions are used but they are disseminated and chosen as solutions to a common problem rather than specified as the only answer.

In order to make use of the worker's ability, they have to know what is required, agree that they wish to make that change and have the ability to make management and appropriate local changes.

Requirements to use this system

- Knowing the aim of the organisation – vision
- A desire to work to improve the service – ownership
- Ability to make change in the hands of the worker – flexibility
- Seeing and acting on the blocks to change – local solutions exploited

There are costs to the individual workers and the business when the environment is very controlling. People have different abilities to work with a defined and controlling system. Where workers do not like the system they can leave.

If the job requires limited training the worker can easily be replaced. If the training is long and costly this is expensive for the business that paid for the training and damaging because the system cannot function without that worker.[30] As jobs have become more skilled, the attitude of the workers has changed and they expect to have some control over their working environment. This now includes many workers not traditionally considered to be professionals.[32] Employers have to adjust to the professionalisation of the whole workforce and change the way they run their businesses to accommodate it. Morale and recruitment will be influenced by the working environment and management style of the employer.[30,32]

Two extremes of management practice exist and any individual organisation is likely to be somewhere in between. At one extreme every detail of job and organisation is managed from above. Everything is specified or micromanaged. At the other extreme, only the bare minimum is specified, which is known as macro-management.

Table 4.1 The relationship between management method and demonstrable management functions.

Measurable management function	Expectation from general management literature (management method)	
	Micro-management	Macro-management
Aim of system known to professionals (vision)	Not required	Required
Ownership of change	Not required	Required
Local solutions exploited	Not required	Required
Flexible systems	No	Yes
Morale and recruitment	Poor	Improved
Overall system efficiency	Poor	Improved

The inter-relationship between the management method and functions enables us to look at any individual organisation and understand which method is being used. We can look at the management methods used within general practice to see if this throws any light on the reasons why change is implemented in some cases but not in apparently similar circumstances where the difference is the personal skills of the managers involved.

There are many things that an individual worker cannot control in a business. There will be skills and structures that involve others that are required some or all of the time. If an organisation has multiple units doing the same thing there is likely to be common experience and systems that would help each individual unit. Running the business becomes a balance between specifying everything to make a system work and allowing local flexibility.

For this reason large companies are moving towards a separation of the workforce. The core team is directly employed and a number of subunits with local autonomy work with the organisation.[32] The central company sets the vision and facilitates the environment of the company by providing the basic framework. It can understand the resources, training and personnel requirements of the whole company. Each subunit plans and understands its local environment and draws on the central resources when it has specific needs such as a fully trained staff member, a new skill requiring training or specialist personnel support for a difficult problem.

General practice is already organised in this devolved manner. It is therefore in a good position to exploit this new thinking.

East Kent Health Authority quality scheme

Description

In order to see if this method works in medicine it was necessary to find a local area where outcome measures were set but process was not defined. It would then be possible to judge whether the method was successful and learn from the methods used to introduce it.

The East Kent Health Authority Primary Care Clinical Effectiveness (PRICCE) scheme does this.[24] It worked with the existing structure of primary care organised as general practices and set clinical outcomes as criteria for quality. The criteria (the parameters that are measured) were selected for each disease area and standards (the level of achievement of that criterion) were set for each criteria. For example, blood pressure will be measured each year in patients with a diagnosis of hypertension (criterion) in 100% of hypertensive patients (standard).

In the PRICCE scheme criteria were selected across 13 major disease areas and very high standards set for the achievement of specific payments. For each criterion there was only one standard. For example, in control of hypertension, the standard was 75% and payment was only made if that level was reached; hence these were target payments. There was no attempt to force particular processes or protocols on the practices. The areas to be included were originally selected by local managers from a group of conditions thought to be evidence based, in areas where the criteria could be as near to the outcome of improved patient care as possible. This aimed to specify the outcome required but leave clinical and managerial freedom to the GPs as the manager responsible for the quality of care provided by the practice. The criteria and standards were discussed with the doctors' representatives for the area (local medical committee) and some small changes made. The criteria and standards which emerged at the end of the process were challenging, in line with or above the best achieved elsewhere for individual diseases for volunteer practices.[33] Once success in all 13 disease areas for every criterion and standard was achieved, the practices received a payment of £3000 per GP per year for an average-sized list. The money was paid in advance but repayable if the targets were not achieved.

There was help with practice development. The normal resources for general practice in the area were available and used for practice development before the project. The practices had buildings, IT support and staff in line with the rest of the NHS before the project. Once it started managers helped with further development of the same type. Additional help specifically for the scheme included facilitation of education meetings and the publication of a booklet of detailed advice. This listed each criterion and standard, the prevalence of the disease and the method to be used to measure it. There was also advice on implementation, which included guidelines that could be used. These were taken from national sources or locally written. Practices were asked to use internal guidelines but which guideline or the source was not specified. There were requirements to enter the scheme: all the GPs had to agree that they wished to participate, they had to be using computers in the consultation room and they had to have conducted at least one audit in the practice. Additional resources were given to a local organisation, the East Kent Medical Audit Advisory Group (MAAG), to help practices understand and achieve the audit requirements of the scheme.

Evaluation of performance

The success of the scheme has prompted much interest. A formal evaluation of the scheme looked at the reasons for its success.[34,35]

Over the first three years of the project, 75% of practices in an entire health authority were facilitated to provide comprehensive chronic disease management. The numbers involved continued to increase after this. True outcomes are difficult to establish and some process measures were chosen instead of true outcomes. For example, changing death rates from ischaemic heart disease would take many years but the proxy of measuring cholesterol and then managing cholesterol to be below 5 mmol/l was used for the scheme. The particular standard for each criterion varied but typically the scheme expected 80% of the entire population to have the parameter measured and 80% of those to have it controlled; this produced results as good as the best schemes looking at individual diseases.[33] The practitioners themselves felt that change had taken place. Exclusions of individuals from the figures were allowed in certain circumstances, including if the patient refused, but many practices did not need to use this option to reach the targets.

The scheme therefore represents a successful local project that used multiple methods together to achieve change. The change was large and implemented across most of an area for multiple diseases at the same time. It is therefore appropriate to look in detail at the reasons for its success.

Features of the scheme leading to success

When asked why they had achieved good results in this particular scheme when they had not performed like this before, the participants said that the scheme provided the following drivers of change:

- improved patient care
- professional pride
- retained autonomy

- additional financial resources
- because they were asked to.

This scheme provided all five drivers of change which allowed individual partners to convince their colleagues that participation was a good idea. Individual GPs were motivated by different factors. The initial questioning of the scheme on clinical grounds was widespread and beneficial. Professionals were challenged to find evidence that meeting the standards was not medically correct.

When they searched the evidence base they educated themselves about the importance of these particular issues. This was important both as a focused educational exercise and later to provide motivation when achieving the criteria proved difficult. Many felt that they were already achieving good results and that the scheme would be relatively easy when they initially entered into it. After their first set of audits they soon found that was not so. However, they had now reviewed the evidence and believed that patients were being harmed if they didn't reach the required levels.

This provided an additional incentive. Motivation often shifted from financial to improving clinical care or professional pride in a job done well. When it became hard, and much additional work was required, the same drivers were important in motivating practices to complete the scheme.

After the scheme, participants also felt that they had changed and were much more committed to providing high-quality chronic disease management. Participants in the scheme were clear that they were trying to improve patient care. Local leaders developed during the process and they have continued to provide clinical leadership. Everyone's feelings of self-worth and morale improved despite the additional work necessary.

The scheme did not specify much organisational change and there were no organisational criteria and standards. Each practice was required to have computers in the consulting room and to have completed an audit and all partners had to agree to work towards the clinical criteria and standards. The managers were aware that development was required but provided resources and advice as their specific managerial input.

The high standards and relatively small resources provided encouraged the practices to use their assets in the most efficient way possible. Each individual practice worked out how to use the staff available to best effect. They used PDSA cycles in the practice to develop local solutions. They were not aware they were doing this but it appeared to be a natural progression to suggest a method of implementing change, try it to see if it worked, if it did keep it, if it didn't look elsewhere. The scheme facilitated access to these ideas for the practices from multiple sources.

The scheme uncovered an educational agenda and focused activity on the scheme. Practitioners went through a specific educational process that started with checking the criteria, finding organisational and clinical gaps in knowledge, using meetings set up by the scheme organisers to share ideas and information. Some also reviewed the evidence base and targeted learning which could be shared with other practices. Internal protocols and guidelines were produced and there was local ownership of these in the practices. Local information sources inside and outside primary care were used. Learners

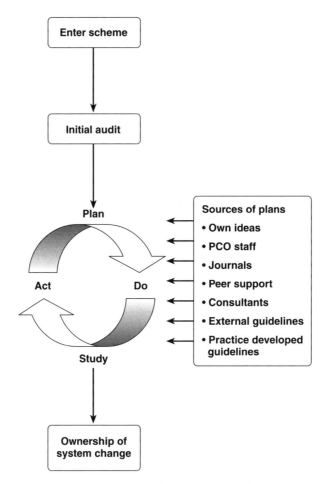

Figure 4.2   Use of PDSA cycles to test and implement external ideas.

described problem-based learning individually and as part of facilitated groups. The increased funding of the MAAG, which was trusted and considered independent by the practices, assisted this.

The criteria and standards of the scheme were summative (pass or fail, like an exam). However, the practices used formative (developmental, like course-work) advice from the MAAG and other sources they found themselves. The practices went looking for possible solutions and tested them by PDSA cycles to see if they worked in their environment. In time the education groups started by the managers became self-sustaining and 'owned' by the clinicians. The individuals who were organising this process became local leaders and were able to help others and lead further development.

Whilst specific organisational change was not required, the managing personnel had a clear intention to develop practices. Spending on IT, premises, staff and staff training were all encouraged. This constituted the specific managerial skill of the managers. New money was found for primary care to pay for the scheme, which sought to exploit the practice-based structure of

GPs to improve care and provided a management focus for the practices. They did not have to work out a public health agenda and long-term plan as this was done for them but they did have to focus their resources on making local changes to succeed.

The reliance on employees to make change happen encouraged practices to value their staff. If the staff produced new methods or implemented their own ways of working the managers or doctors accepted this and allowed them increasing autonomy. The quality of teams and delegation increased. The staff described ownership of the task and a desire to succeed in improving patient care. Some individuals resisted change, didn't use teams and worked harder. They were allowed to do so but in the end understood the need for change and created their own team-working solutions.

Once the standards were met the individuals within the practices displayed a pride in their achievement. Their morale was improved as a result of the process. Practices felt they had worked hard to achieve the change and a few felt they had personally gained financially. The increased resource was used to pay for more staff and equipment. The GPs' and their employees' view of chronic disease management changed as a result of the scheme. They felt that managing all their patients, even those who were non-compliant or lost in the system, was important.

There were some negative impacts. The scheme proved so effective in achieving its aims that it focused care away from patients. It used a great many doctor appointments for chronic disease management. It was not possible to achieve the whole change through nurse-run clinics. Patient-initiated appointments became more difficult to obtain. The GPs did not feel that patient care suffered but time to appointment lengthened as the GPs were overseeing a different and new task. The scheme achieved major change with no increase in GP numbers. If the old task, reactive patient care, was to be achieved as well GP numbers would have needed to increase or the new task, systematic care of illness, further delegated.

The PRICCE scheme used targets. There was only one level of perform-ance that would achieve success and practices had to achieve these high standards across all 13 disease areas to keep the financial payments. When they discovered how much work was involved they reconsidered whether they wished to complete the project, using the same drivers to decide if they wished to continue. Individual motivation did change. There was change between drivers, some from income motivation to one of quality or pride in a job done well, whilst others worked hard to avoid repaying money.

This second cycle and the further work were important in achieving the high standards of the project. It is possible to see that these forced practices to concentrate on this area of work and may have influenced the negative aspects of the scheme of concentration on the targets to the exclusion of other work.

The scheme involved 75% of practices by the third wave. By the end of the third year of the scheme, audited data existed showing uniformly high levels of management for these 13 diseases. Other practices were still agreeing to participate in different ways or in the full scheme. Variability between practices was markedly reduced and the health authority and its successor body, the PCO, knew which practices were not achieving the criteria and

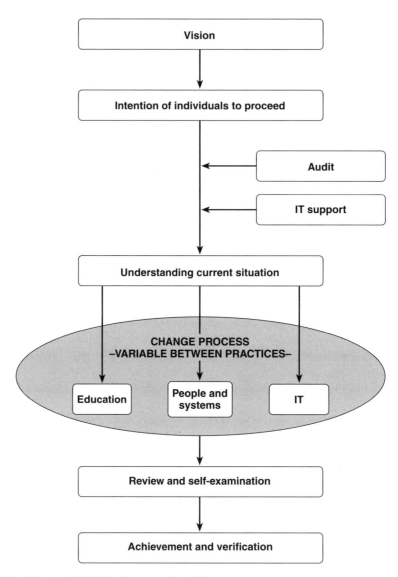

Figure 4.3 How the PRICCE scheme produced change.

standards. Investigation and resources could now be used to find out why a much smaller number of practices were not succeeding and help them to improve. Practices in the first and second wave were interviewed and accepted that variation had reduced and care was more systematic. Managers were confident that variation was much reduced.

There were a small number of practices that could not achieve the targets. Improvement occurred in all. Of the two interviewed (the total number at that time), one later achieved the targets and the other was unhappy with the inability to access resources without reaching the target level itself but was proud of the improvement achieved.

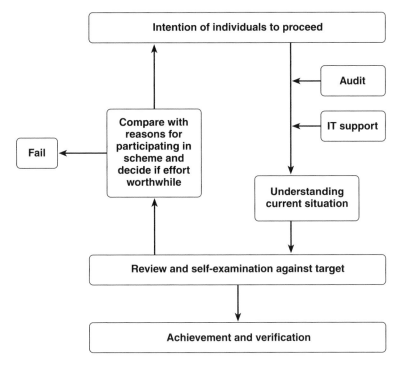

Figure 4.4 Effect of targets on the implementation of standards.

The evaluation attempted to find out why some practices were not participating. Practices that were unhappy with the scheme were working on the same clinical areas and improving care despite not entering the scheme and not receiving the additional resources. The reasons given for declining to participate in the scheme were also related to the drivers for the scheme. They described a feeling of reduced autonomy (because the scheme specified aspects of care) and a feeling that concentrating on chronic care would damage acute reactive patient care and availability. Ultimately the numbers proved small but enforcing particular patterns of care will have an effect on individuals.

Conclusion

The promulgation of guidelines by many individual methods has not produced change.[23] There is evidence that increasing control over practitioners reduces involvement and increases burnout.[28] This increased control is implicated in the decision of some GPs to leave the service.

Outcome-based targets in specific clinical areas and managed in a specific way produced rapid beneficial change in multiple diseases over the majority of a health authority population.

Using outcomes to set criteria and standards and monitor success does not solve all the problems of attempting to focus improvement on a particular

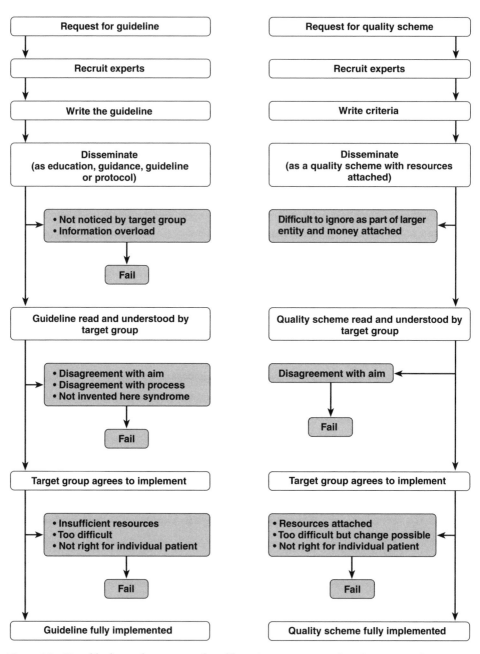

Figure 4.5 How blocks to change are reduced by using outcomes rather than protocols.

area. They can be used to avoid reducing autonomy by leaving the methods to be used for change to the practice. It remains true that the method still requires the professional to perform a particular externally defined change. Most of the problems in Figure 4.1 are no longer an issue but some remain and limit the use of the technique.

If the clinicians do not feel the change is clinically appropriate then it will still be difficult to implement, whether in the form of a protocol or scheme. The detail and form of the criteria and standards in a scheme are important.

Box 4.2 Clinicians have to believe the intervention will work before they will implement it

Example: implementing a stop smoking strategy[36]

A health promotion payment was created for practices when clinicians changed patient behaviour to stop smoking. The clinicians did not believe the specific intervention of confronting patients about smoking in consultations about other unrelated matters was appropriate. Behaviour did not change although, for some, recording and claiming improved for work already performed.

Where clinicians feel the specific intervention requested is clinically incorrect, even if autonomy and the overall purpose are accepted, it will not be implemented.

The East Kent scheme is written as a contract. It therefore provides understanding of a different method of implementation and a method of turning change management into a contract. A contract in this context implies a written agreement between the employing authority and the practice, specifying what will be achieved by the practice for the provision of defined resources or rewards from the employer. The specification of quality as a series of criteria and standards is a requirement for use in a contractual setting.

The specification of financial payments for specific criteria and standards is relatively easy. The structure of the scheme implies that by specifying a limited number of criteria, autonomy of method for those criteria is left to the practice. These managers gave autonomy to the practices and honoured that part of the contract even when practices wanted to go their own way. Provided they succeeded in meeting the criteria and standards, they were allowed to use different methods. The managerial method also needs to be replicated for success elsewhere.

The reaction in practices is similar to the macro-management model described for general management. The effects are shown in Table 4.2.

When the scheme is a priority for the clinical unit involved, guidelines and process measures no longer need to be forced on clinicians as they then look for practical methods to achieve the scheme. The relationship to guidelines changes and the practices go looking for information. Guidelines and information from authoritative organisations (e.g. NICE, SIGN, British Hypertension Society) should be made available which then become positive sources of help to the participants in a scheme. Process measures then follow the attitudinal change of wanting to achieve the criteria. High standards in multiple areas oblige methods to change to achieve them. Working harder cannot do it. Eventually participants realise they should work smarter. Therefore working methods change to solve the problems in the individual practice. Development occurs and capacity is created for further change.

Table 4.2 Table showing how the PRICCE scheme and guideline implementation differ in their use of management functions and the similarities
with management methods in the general management literature.

	Expectation from general management literature		Central organisation and creation of process	East Kent experience
Management function	Micro-management	Macro-management	Promotion of guidelines	Fixed outcomes Devolved process
Aim of system known to professionals (vision)	Not required	Required	Yes	Yes
Ownership of change	Not required	Required	No	Yes
Local solutions exploited	Not required	Required	No	Yes
Flexible systems	No	Yes	No	Adapted to one change; no long-term experience
Morale and recruitment	Poor	Improved	? Reduced	Morale improved after success

Chapter 5

Other quality improvement methods used in medicine

Quality schemes

A number of quality schemes have been developed, initially by professional organisations interested in quality and latterly by some primary care groups (PCG) and trusts (PCT). Usually a group from the host organisation produces a list of important areas that would benefit from review and develops criteria to assess each area. Some of the criteria are summative and require data to be produced to show that specific standards have been achieved. For example, summaries of medical records will be produced and will be available for 90% of patients. Other criteria are formative, where the practice is expected to think about an issue and produce its own solution to the problem, which is written down as part of a submission. For example, the practice will produce a list of rules to enable summaries to be produced. By using a combination of summative and formative assessments across a number of areas, a picture of the practice can be built up.

Box 5.1 An example quality scheme

Quality Practice Award (QPA)[37]

An award run by the Royal College of General Practitioners (RCGP) for practices. The practice has to produce written evidence to demonstrate it has achieved criteria and standards organised into 17 different areas of practice. The criteria are a mix of formative and summative. Most practices entering the scheme would meet some criteria but require effort to meet all criteria. The process encourages them to improve all practice systems up to a high standard and reduce the variability of internal systems.

The evidence is reviewed by a team of three assessors drawn from GPs, practice managers, practice nurses and lay visitors. If the written evidence is satisfactory the practice is visited by the team and the evidence reviewed in the practice. Some criteria require physical checking on the day, for example that the notes are correctly summarised, and others by speaking to the GPs and staff. The formative assessments are reviewed with colleagues and further thinking and development discussed. In this way the detail of practice organisation is subjected to peer review.

As the award is for the practice, it does not examine individual clinical work but does look in detail at organisation, practice systems and planning.

The practices volunteer to participate and are seeking to change. The status of the awards is high and the practices are willing to put in substantial amounts of work to achieve an award. Professionals attending the practice to discuss formative criteria and how they were developed gain an overview of the way the practice works and can discuss good and less good areas of practice. Even in areas without specific criteria, the assessors can request information. The practice can use this as a method of finding out how they compare to others, a form of benchmarking.

Quality schemes of this type are available for individual practitioners, including Membership by Assessment of Performance (MAP) and Fellowship by Assessment (FBA) from the RCGP. Practices can gain the Quality Team Development and Quality Practice Award from the RCGP. Practice and other managers can achieve Fellowship by Assessment of the Institute of Healthcare Management. The Health Quality Service has a primary care module and similar schemes for assessment in secondary care.

The act of producing their own guidelines and auditing their own practice develops new skills and is beneficial. The practice has access to a local supporter when preparing for the assessment. The practice has to make changes before it is assessed as the standard required on the day is defined. Schemes are thought to produce favourable change and participants rate them highly as positive experiences which lead to change which benefits patients. Participants do not have the negative reactions seen when external control agendas are enforced. Formative criteria allow autonomy to the practice up to a point. If poor medical practice is found that falls below General Medical Council (GMC) or Nursing and Midwifery Council (NMC) standards then action is expected.

Inspections of this type require assessors who will be respected by participants. This necessitates the use of professionals from the same peer group. Assessments require a great deal of preparation of written material and practice change before the visit. The review of the written evidence and the visit itself take considerable time from highly skilled assessors. Some of the awards are subsidised but the cost in replacement time and opportunity cost of the professionals' time is large.

Other existing NHS structures

Modernisation Agency

This agency was established to assist managers and professionals with change. The published aims are in line with TQM and espouse local development and local ownership of problems and solutions. This could encompass a number of methods of working but specific methods are currently being used.

The Modernisation Agency has funded facilitators to help practices with specific projects. An example of this is advanced access.

Box 5.2 Implementing TQM principles by implementing processes

Example: advanced access[38]

Here the aim is to reduce the length of wait for a GP appointment.

Initial work in practices and PDSA cycles showed that a particular method would reduce appointment waits. A local facilitator is appointed and provides help and support to practices to audit their appointment system. The practice audits to find out how many appointments are required for each day of the week. Change is made to increase appointments or divert demand. The practice only makes appointments available one day in advance. The practice sees the backlog of patients on a one-off basis as extra work but, once done, the practice can stay in balance and provide appointments. There are funds available to help with the initial work of reducing the backload, which can be variable between practices.

If there are enough appointments the system works well. If there are not enough appointments the number needs to be increased or patients diverted to phone calls or other members of the team whether they want that or not. Appointments far into the future are reduced.

As described earlier for TQM, the solution is worked out in one setting and the method implemented elsewhere with local support and some flexibility.

In this change management programme, a single topic is chosen, the practice is encouraged or helped to audit their own current performance and specific audit tools are available. The practice is then asked to review its performance against benchmark norms and encouraged to work out methods to improve performance. Specific solutions are available plus a small amount of resource to overcome any local factors stopping change.

In a general practice setting the facilitator is employed for more than one practice and becomes an external agent of change in one area of interest to the practice. The practice is still required to find human resources and solutions to an idea focused on by the initiative. The initiative works to induce change in one area of medicine at one time.

Whilst there could be a number of simultaneous initiatives there is no incentive to make fundamental changes to working methods to solve the whole problem faced by the practice. Multiple initiatives may well result in disparate requests for change and conflicting solutions.

The existing structure of general practices, with relatively small independent units, fits better with incentives to produce local solutions to a specification for the whole practice. The existing practice accreditation schemes do this by providing a peer-led facilitated intervention to tackle all areas of practice development at once.

Government initiatives to standardise healthcare

NICE was created to give opinions on best practice.[19,20] It is responsible for these activities in England and Wales and reviews evidence and publishes evidence-based guidance. SIGN was originally founded in 1993 as a professional organisation and creates definitive evidence-based guidelines in Scotland. These government agencies are charged with advising government and the professions on the appropriateness of technologies, treatments and medical practice.

They produce guidance on how to achieve outcomes or what to use. They are not themselves charged with implementation. They produce detailed evidence and advice and a ready source of authoritative information. Change management schemes can use them as a source of detailed toolkits and resources for use as a secondary change method.

NSFs have been produced for areas the government wishes to prioritise and aim to standardise the service. They only apply to England and Wales; Scotland has a different set of National Priorities which perform the same function. They apply to primary and secondary care and detail the level of care that is expected. They are intended to be used as service planning documents when services are commissioned. The cost of the staff required to implement the priorities and their training is calculated as part of the framework. NSFs vary in style and content. Some, for example diabetes and cardiovascular NSFs, contain detailed lists of services to be provided to patients. Others, for example mental health and care of the elderly, have broad concepts and few specific requirements.

NSFs and National Priorities have implications for cost in the NHS. If a provision to do something exists it has to be achieved and paid for. The number of provisions that relate to primary care varies between NSFs and National Priorities. The priorities expressed in these documents are important for the PCOs in the four UK countries and they are responsible for delivering the plans. These priorities were not available when the old GMS contract was published but some have been incorporated into PMS contracts at local level.

Clinical governance is the mechanism used to implement the NSFs and National Priorities in NHS trusts.[20] The trust has to ensure that its staff carry out priorities of the respective health services, using the guidelines from NICE and SIGN. This is to be developmental and supportive in helping professionals to understand and implement change. Each organisation, in this case the practice, is to have a professional development plan that lists development priorities for the next year. That plan is accomplished by the individuals within the practice and the same tasks are used to create the personal development plans of the practice clinicians and managers. The aim is a uniform service with all services provided to an equal and high standard across the country. Each NHS trust is accountable for its clinical governance. Poor practice is to be dealt with by professional self-regulation. For a doctor this means the poorly performing doctor procedures of the GMC. There are equivalent procedures for other clinicians involving their own professional organisations.

An inspectorate achieves accountability to the governments. CHI inspects NHS trusts to check whether clinical governance arrangements are satisfactory.[20]

The methods for reviewing PCTs focus on the patient experience, strategic management capacity, health improvement and securing service delivery, together with the seven components of clinical governance.[39]

- Patient, service user, carer and public involvement
- Risk management
- Clinical audit
- Staffing and management
- Education and training
- Clinical effectiveness
- Use of information.

CHI is also charged with investigating poor performance and errors. It is soon to be replaced by the Commission for Health Audit and Inspection (CHAI) which is similar but has additional audit responsibilities.

Conclusion

Local quality schemes introduced by professional bodies have produced change but do not lead to comparable standards and are expensive if the full cost of professional time is taken into account. Formative assessments are generally well received by participants. The existing structure of general practice, of small units, favours review of multiple areas in one practice at one time.

The principles of local development using PDSA cycles are promoted by government agencies as the way forward. They have worked well in specific areas. There is a requirement to broaden this method to other areas. The difference between the TQM approach followed by the Modernisation Agency and an outcome-based scheme is the level of autonomy open to the practice to make changes to the expected solution locally.

The detail of the best schemes can be used to create other schemes in other areas of medicine or for the new GP contract. This can be created in practices by using a series of criteria and allowing and encouraging the practice to find a solution. The cost of the scheme will vary depending on whether formative or summative criteria are used. Any method that requires formative change will require more time and hence cost.

Chapter 6

Designing a quality improvement scheme

Overall scheme design

Using the principles of the work in the quality schemes, it is possible to design a scheme that would produce change in different areas of medicine. The overall structure of the scheme itself should provide the drivers of autonomy, professional pride, resources and clear requests for action. Each individual criterion should provide improved patient care. The choice of the criteria affects whether the five drivers are present.

The scheme needs to provide:

- Autonomy
- Professional pride
- Resources
- Clear request for action

Each criterion needs to provide:

- Improved patient care

Table 6.1 Designing the five drivers into a scheme.

Driver	How designed into the contract
Improving patient care	Select important clinical criteria accepted by participants as improving care of patients (carefully chosen criteria)
Autonomy	Allow autonomy of process within supported structures with stated boundaries
Professional pride	Encourage professionals to help with creating and monitoring the task against values shared by the group. True devolution of the task is required to allow the professionals to shape the task over time. The highest levels need to be challenging and allow pride and recognition for achievement
Resources	Create a financial arrangement that reflects the work and costs involved in the task so the resources (people and systems) themselves can be employed and used
Clear request for action	Clarity about the nature of the task required and the format of the description and assessment method to make the requirements precise

The scheme consists of a series of criteria and standards that describe what is to be achieved. Achievement of the criteria is assessed and the success recognised. This could be an award, e.g. Quality Practice Award, or it could be a financial payment. It could be a single payment for the whole scheme or multiple stepped payments for achievement. The payment could be a reward for completion of a task to a high level or be used to purchase more people and systems to assist in achieving the task.

It would be possible to structure the reward as access to staff or equipment from outside without any need for financial payment. This would reduce the autonomy available as the employer or provider of the additional resource would influence the clinical unit.

Designing clinical criteria

It is important to create a method that can be applied to new areas. In order to do this there needs to be a stepwise process for the creation of criteria to fit with an overall scheme for the area of medicine that is being targeted. A number of thought processes are required which are summarised in Box 6.1. Each phase is explored to enable criteria to be written in different areas.

Box 6.1 Outline of the process used to create criteria and standards

- Choose the area of medicine to target
- Select important issues within that area that professionals will accept to improve care
- Decide on a measurement method (formative or summative)
- Look for evidence of current best practice in the area
- Formulate as a series of criteria
- Moderate the criteria to increase the population to be measured (indicators or audit criteria)
- Check if measurement is possible and decide on a method
- Set standard
- Decide on data collection method
- Design or develop IT or other system to facilitate data collection
- Design a reporting and assessment system
- Train assessors

In reality most of the stages are considered as a single entity when creating criteria. If something can't be measured there is little point in doing the preparatory work of formulating the criterion. However, it is important that the quality improvement is the driver for writing the criterion rather than the ability to measure it. Choosing criteria that are easy to measure or using available information simply because it is routinely collected is likely to damage the quality improvement scheme.

General considerations for writing criteria

This method can be used in other areas of medicine or specialist practice if criteria can be found that are acceptable within a scheme. It is first necessary to consider the area or specialty to be measured and find appropriate criteria to use. Whichever area of medicine is involved, the criteria chosen need to improve outcomes for the patients. A similar unit of a small number of clinicians and supporting staff is appropriate for a similar approach. The term 'clinical unit' is used in the description and the examples are all from a general practice setting.

For change to occur as a result of setting a criterion, the clinical unit has to be able to produce change. Criteria should be selected that the clinical unit can control and achieve.

In order to recreate the overall scheme design, the clinical unit should be given outcomes to aim for. The difficulty in finding true outcomes means that process measures as near to outcomes as possible are used instead. For example, the outcome measure might be a reduction in premature mortality and the chosen measure would be control of high blood pressure, cholesterol or smoking. Once clinicians were persuaded that the individual criteria were appropriate, they would want to find out how they are performing personally. This will give ownership of the task and involvement in the outcome of the project. This will only happen if the clinicians believe that achieving the criteria will improve patient care.

The criteria selected should also measure the factors that make a big difference, not every minor aspect of care. For example, checking the measurement of urea and electrolytes within one week of starting an ACE inhibitor is good practice but too detailed to use in a general practice setting. If important clinical criteria are chosen then the benefit of any particular criterion must be achieved. For example, the measurement and control of blood pressure is important and, if achieved, will improve morbidity and mortality.

It is important to improve patient care and reduce gaming (the ability to achieve apparent success but not improve care). If a marker of care is chosen alone, say number of patients on a waiting list, then that can improve but other important issues like the length of wait or the waiting time for more serious problems can rise even though the standard is achieved. Clinical criteria are more likely to meet this requirement than organisational criteria. Well-chosen criteria that are important to patient care are less likely to result in gaming.

Improving patient care for the whole population is important. Those lost to follow-up or reluctant to attend should be included in the population measured. When a small unit is involved it is possible to set up systems to measure the whole population with a particular illness. If the small unit is patients with a specific illness, say renal failure, in a PCO area it is important for the database to be comprehensive and include all patients whether attending the unit or looked after elsewhere. Therefore an accurate disease register for the population to be measured must be available or possible. The patient data remain with the clinical unit or practice and production of data requires the inclusion of every patient on registers and ultimately treatment.

In order to utilise the strengths of the clinical unit to change treatment, the data have to be available inside the clinical unit. The data should be in a format that allows staff to find the patients and decide who are missing certain interventions. This will require a searchable computer database. It is important when designing criteria to remember that criteria should be amenable to local data collection.

If the data to be collected are used in patient care already, they can be entered as part of routine work. This will be helpful to those required to enter and collect the data. Data already collected in a clinical environment are likely to relate to the important aspects of care. Data collected outside the clinical environment for other reasons may not be appropriate.

Choose criteria that:

- Apply to the population in which they are used
- Can be changed by the clinical unit
- Measure outcomes
- Reflect macro-management not micro-management
- Improve patient care directly
- Apply to whole populations
- Have available clinical data in the clinical unit

Practices or other small units within medicine have to develop the infra-structure to support improved performance. For example, the availability and use of information technology or the employment and training of staff can be specified as criteria. Linking financial resources and payments to the provision of organisational structure allows resources to be made available as cost and complexity increase. The ideas of clinicians and managers in the most developed clinical units can be used by less developed ones to guide their development. It is more difficult to set outcomes to achieve improvement without specifying how the developing unit should organise itself and there-fore criteria often specify processes. For example, requiring the practice to have internal policies can standardise and improve care. Unfortunately, requiring the presence of internal policies is easily 'gamed' by taking some off the shelf and producing them for assessment without impacting on the way the practice is run.

For organisational criteria there is a balance to be struck between requiring specific internal management strategies that remove choice and autonomy and requesting actions that may not produce real change.

Clinical staff are governed by professional codes of conduct. These, along with legal requirements, lend themselves to use as organisational criteria. They are a baseline requirement and have to be implemented by all. The formulation of professional codes that list minimum and best practice, for example *Good Medical Practice for GPs*, allows a progression of development. For example this publication specifies that notes should be comprehensive, legible and completed for every consultation. This can be used to create a baseline requirement and organisational criteria.

The most important organisational tasks for a clinical unit can be identified. These are the ones that would result in frequent or catastrophic failure if they were not present. The criteria themselves reflect an agreed way to proceed that specifies the essential part of the task but leaves other aspects that do not need to be closely defined for local implementation. This process is assisted by working out why there was a need to specify a particular way to proceed. Changing the measurement method can help with this problem of enforcing single solutions to development challenges.

If the scheme is to apply to a clinical unit there will be staff employed by the unit who are not directly involved in managing the quality scheme. There is a requirement to treat staff well and meet good employment practice. For example, all staff should have job descriptions.

When criteria are set and clinical data are used to prove quality there is a requirement for the clinician to enter all readings and to enter them honestly. No method will prove that every reading is accurate. Clinicians are expected to be honest about those parameters that they directly measure or record. There are many opportunities to measure parameters and it will become obvious if incorrect readings are used. Speaking to staff, asking to see policies and measuring outcomes all triangulate between the different criteria and will give a wider picture of the unit involved.

In addition, any individual who is willing to enter incorrect data is just as likely to enter false results or not record the data at all. Clinicians enter the medical profession to treat patients. If clinically appropriate criteria are chosen that clinicians believe will improve clinical outcomes, they will be powerfully motivated to enter data correctly and improve treatment.

Decide on a measurement method (formative or summative)

When a scheme is produced it is necessary to be able to measure the criteria. This is done by setting standards for the criteria selected. The way the criteria are written will be affected by the way they will be measured. The nature of the assessment has to be considered early in the development process. Measurement of some criteria demands greater skills or peer group assessment. They also take much more time from the assessor and the assessed than others.

Formative assessment schemes

If the standards are designed to allow latitude and encourage the internal development of processes to achieve change then a formative process will occur. Criteria are designed and written in such a way as to encourage learning and development for those to be assessed. This is presented to the assessor as the equivalent of marked coursework.

This requires criteria to be written in a flexible way. Participants in a scheme can be asked to think about an issue and produce a piece of work, usually a written description, to demonstrate that they have looked at the subject and created a local solution. If the criterion is well written it will focus attention on previous performance and improvement. It is possible to require the achievement of a standard or the production of the development work alone could be sufficient.

Box 6.2   Designing a formative criterion

A formative criterion could be:

'The practice will produce a policy to answer the phone.'

This could result in a detailed review of the telephone system, the standards required and the systems to produce a good service. Alternatively, in the absence of an endpoint or standard, this could be met by writing something which is very easy to achieve and worthless.

'A single receptionist will answer the phone when it is convenient between other work.'

The criterion will have been met but little achieved. Therefore the criteria are made more specific.

'The practice will produce a policy to answer the phone in four rings or less.'

There can be considerable advantages to this process but there could also be difficulties. Most of these advantages and disadvantages would apply for individual formative criteria within a scheme. Where a criterion is reviewed by assessors who are peers there can be detailed discussion of the policies suggested which leads to further change. The achievement of one of these schemes brings professional recognition. As the practice can write its own policies to meet the criteria, it retains the ability to make its own decisions and have autonomy over the method used to meet the criterion.

Some clinical decisions are easy but others require judgement and there is no obvious correct clinical pathway. If investigations are to be targeted there is a need for judgement. Detailed discussion with peers can explore clinical decision making and challenge assumptions. Several techniques have been developed to aid understanding.

Box 6.3   A technique to assess one aspect of clinical care

For example, in Fellowship by Assessment of the RCGP, delay pattern analysis looks at the process and length of time to diagnose a particular illness. A detailed description of five cases with, say, bowel cancer is presented and discussed with colleagues. In addition, video tapes of 10 consecutive consultations are examined and discussed with peers. Detailed formative assessment allows clinical decisions to be examined.

Most of the disadvantages are created by the same issues. The flexibility in the method used to achieve the formative criteria is agreed with the assessor. Consequently there is the possibility that the standard will be different in different practices. Volunteers for peer group review are likely to have a different attitude. The greatest benefit will be obtained if the clinician is open and brings difficult situations for review. Some of the techniques, such as delay pattern analysis and video (*see* Box 6.3), can be chosen to show the best cases. The assessment cannot be detailed and yet apply to the whole population.

The existing schemes are constantly developing and criteria are changed on a regular basis. If the scheme were being relied on to assess a specific area, the development over time could leave out that specific area. Conversely, if the scheme is unchanged, repeating the scheme will assess the same criteria with similar evidence. This will produce further data but because formative change has occurred, further change by repeating the same criteria may not produce sufficient further change to justify the work involved. It may be more helpful to move on to a different area of medicine. Peer group assessment is labour intensive. If clinicians are assessing others they cannot be doing their original jobs. Even if finance were available to pay for a replacement, the number of appropriately skilled clinicians available for participation in assessment is limited.

Advantages of formative quality schemes

- Detailed peer inspection
- Formative process leading to cultural change
- Professional recognition of achievement
- Autonomy retained by practice within limits
- Clinical decision making can be examined
- Volunteers strive to improve
- Process not defined

Disadvantages of formative quality schemes

- Standard reached can be variable
- Compulsion to enter may result in hidden data
- Content can change to be inappropriate
- Capacity difficulties in applying to all practices at one time
- Repetition of the same quality scheme is less likely to produce change with each iteration

---

Summative assessment schemes

A different method of designing criteria uses the criterion and a standard to specify exactly what is required. No attempt is made to discuss how development occurred; it is simply a measurement that is pass or fail. It is the equivalent of the traditional exam.

> **Box 6.4** Designing a summative criterion and standard
>
> In the example of answering the telephone used earlier:
>
> 'The telephone will be answered in four rings or less for 70% of calls.'

This can then be used in exactly the same way in many different sites. It is easier to assess and does not require peers to comment for assessment. If the practice does not meet the standard it still has to change to reach the required level. If it has failed it may well benefit from engaging in a formative process.

Advantages of summative quality schemes

- Criteria and standards reached are fixed
- Same level for all participants
- Repetition of the same quality scheme produces the same result each time
- Professional recognition of achievement
- Autonomy retained by the practice within limits

Disadvantages of summative quality schemes

- No detailed peer inspection
- Measurement but no formative process leading to cultural change
- Clinical decision making not examined
- For some criteria large amounts of process are fixed as guidance on interpretation of criteria

Combined assessment, formative and summative

It is entirely possible to combine the two methods. This is often done in the commonly used schemes. For example, a criterion might read: 'The practice will produce a policy to answer the phone in four rings or less. This will be audited and achieved'.

Look for evidence of current best practice in the area

This requires reviewing the evidence and current best practice. It is appropriate to review individual papers or authoritative sources. Where available, NICE guidance and NSFs (England and Wales) and SIGN guidance and National Priorities (Scotland) are helpful. There is a need to check that the research evidence applies to the area of medicine concerned. For example, much research work is carried out in selected populations with multiple illnesses excluded. It may apply to general populations with multiple illnesses or it may not. Similarly, techniques that work well in general populations with low levels of illness may not apply to specialist populations previously selected for a particular characteristic.

There will not always be evidence for every clinical activity. Even if the evidence is clear there may be an element of choice on the part of the patient. This limits the ability to set summative criteria for that area.

The evidence and the criteria produced need to be acceptable to the clinicians who are to implement the scheme. There are many other stakeholders in the change process. It is also necessary to have credible criteria for other interested parties in the change process. For example, the criteria for a local NHS scheme in general practice would need to be credible to the commissioners of the project (PCO), local managers, consultants for the specialties concerned and patients.

Formulate as criteria

This requires a clear and unambiguous statement of what is to be measured. This varies slightly depending on the payment method for achieving the criterion. Criteria are usually written in the form of something that has been done. They assume complete achievement and state what will be achieved. This is then moderated by the proportion of the population for which they are to be achieved – the standard.

If the reward is for a stepped achievement, say 70%, 80% or 90%, then there is a target. Similarly, if achieving a criterion results in a professional award or recognition at a particular level, then there is a target to aim for.

If a target payment for reaching a set level is envisaged this is all that is required; for example, 'blood pressure will be measured annually in hypertensive patients (standard of 80%)'. If a sliding scale of payment is expected with increasing reward for increasing achievement then the proportionate achievement is the starting point; for example, 'the proportion of hypertensive patients with blood pressure measured in the last year'.

In all cases the criterion must clearly and unambiguously state what is required.

A clinical area can be large and in order to make criteria clear it is necessary to use two or more to describe what is to be achieved. Often three levels of criteria are required: structure, process and outcome. There is a requirement to produce a disease register (structure), to measure a particular parameter (process) and to control that parameter to a specified level (outcome). Long lists of parameters to check are difficult to assess so it is better to use one criterion for one assessment.

The nature of the evidence usually helps to guide the wording of criteria. It is necessary to state what is to be measured in which population and how often. If the measurement is to be audited it is easier to specify the recording process as part of the criterion. The criteria should be short enough to understand the essence of what is to be measured. Other definitions and detailed guidance can be added as supporting documentation.

Box 6.5 An example of writing multiple criteria for a disease area (diabetes)

'The practice will produce an accurate register of diabetes mellitus patients.'

Once the register is available relevant parameters can be measured.

'Patients with diabetes mellitus should have their HbA1c recorded every 12 months.'

Once the HbA1c has been measured it is important to fix an outcome measure. In diabetes, current best practice is an HbA1c of 7 or below, leading to a criterion of:

'In diabetes mellitus patients the recorded HbA1c will be 7 or below.'

If a criterion is asking for something to be done in a new way that could not have been expected before, it is appropriate to give a start date. This is a prospective criterion. This avoids setting criteria that are impossible to meet; for example, 'patients who suffer a myocardial infarction should have a cholesterol level taken within six weeks'. If the myocardial infarction was three years ago there is no possibility of meeting the criterion for that patient. Even if the activity was good practice at the time it cannot be changed and the aim is to improve care in the future.

Words mean what words say when written as criteria. They need to be examined for unexpected meanings that either undermine the criterion or introduce incentives to inappropriate practice. A good criterion is one that sufficiently tightly specifies what is to be measured and measures it in a standard way to a standard level. Unexpected problems emerge after writing and therefore it is better to observe how criteria are used and what problems arise before trying to 'fix' criteria. Most schemes gradually develop criteria and audit methods for this reason.

Criteria need to be developed and it is much easier to use or adapt existing criteria.

Moderate to increase the population to be measured: creating indicators or audit criteria

When evidence is collected to improve medicine there is an aim to be at the leading edge of practice and to show what can be achieved. Initially the populations are selected to try to measure one parameter alone. For any given parameter, say the treatment of diabetes mellitus, studies could be done with the aim of achieving different levels in different trials, say HbA1c of 8 in one and 7 in another. Over time multiple trials will suggest a treatment level which is usually then turned into guidance at a specific treatment level; for example, HbA1c should be controlled to below 7, as in the English NSF.

Whilst this is good practice, it is accepted that the constraints of treatment methodology and real patients mean that it can only be achieved for a proportion of patients, say 40%. It follows that criteria and standards have to be set with this in mind. There is therefore a choice between setting tight criteria and low standards or looser criteria and high standards. In order to achieve the greatest improvement in healthcare, the largest number of patients should be included in the audited population.

Managing diabetes is difficult and high and low readings of the HbA1c measure different things. Therefore a higher audit criterion is required, say 7.4. This is only likely to apply to a proportion of the population, say 50%. Some properly advised and treated patients will have a higher HbA1c than this. They should not, however, have very high levels, say above 10. This would arise in an uncontrolled situation. There might be good clinical or social reasons for a small number but most should be below this level, say 90%. Therefore two audit criteria with different standards are required for the same parameter to show good treatment for a moderate proportion and reasonable treatment for the vast majority.

'In diabetes mellitus patients the recorded HbA1c will be 7 or below.'
'In diabetes mellitus patients the recorded HbA1c will be 10 or below.'

In addition, some measurements, for example blood pressure, are subject to variation about a mean level. For example, if the average blood pressure is 138/84 on any given day, a proportion of readings will be lower and some higher. If all readings were to be below the level originally set as an average then the mean blood pressure would have to be lower still. In the practical situation of blood pressure control for a population there has to be a limit on the number of blood pressures that can be recorded for an individual in the reporting period. However, if the blood pressure is measured annually and the reading is high there is no ability to control that blood pressure by changing medication or other method. Consequently the criterion has to be set at a level above the best achievable practice and the time interval for the audit set longer than the expected measurement cycle.

Box 6.6 An example of moderating an evidence-based criterion to increase the number of patients in the assessment

For blood pressure, expected best practice is less than 140/85 measured annually (realistic expectation of standard 50%)
Audit is carried out at less than or equal to 150/90 on readings in the last 15 months (realistic expectation of standard 80%)

This is sometimes called an audit standard but this term is confusing. It is properly known as an audit criterion. It is also called an indicator, which could also be taken to mean a proxy measure for something else, say the measurement of the proportion of medicines prescribed generically as an indicator of prescribing quality. This is not meant here. An indicator is a way of writing a criterion to enable it to be used for audit purposes.

The way this is applied and the leeway available to do this for individual criteria vary. For some indicators, lowering the mean to achieve a tight criterion is unequivocally a good thing but for others it is not. For example, reducing the mean blood pressure well below 140/85 to make all readings below 140/85 would probably lead to a number of patients with unacceptably low blood pressure and symptomatic problems. However, the lowering of cholesterol below an accepted treatment level would not result in more morbidity because the side effects of the medication and treating the condition do not increase in this situation. Therefore the setting of audit criteria requires judgement and the margin between best practice and the audit criteria will vary between criteria.

The level and amount of difference required will depend on the amount of variation about the mean for each individual parameter. The number of readings affects this. There is a mathematical relationship between the mean and standard deviations for any given parameter governed by the amount of variation in the parameter and the measurement method. For practical reasons, and to allow change to occur in a parameter, the single last reading has to be used. This is to allow change to occur. Otherwise a single high reading (real) followed by treatment at one year and a real reduction would not achieve the audit standard within the 15-month audit period.

Box 6.7 Effect of averaging blood pressure readings with defined measurement intervals

Scenario

A patient with a previously controlled blood pressure attending for an annual review. The criterion is systolic blood pressure 150 or below.

Reading 1 at 1 year	170
2 weeks later	175
2 weeks later (Rx increased)	170
2 weeks later	160
2 weeks later	160
2 weeks later (Rx increased)	165
2 weeks later	140

Now 15 months – no more readings allowed

Average of the last three results (155) – criterion not met
Last result (140) – criterion met

Averaging the last three BP readings makes it difficult to demonstrate control in a short period of time, especially if it takes repeated changes of medication to achieve BP control.

Check if measurement is possible and decide on a method

There are many areas of medicine that could be agreed by most clinicians as good practice but are difficult or impossible to measure. Summative criteria require a reliable and reproducible measurement method. This is partly a function of the area of clinical medicine. There is a measurement for cholesterol. A scale could be used for fatigue or pain but it is inherently more difficult. If there is a measurement then a summative criterion can be used. It is possible to change what is monitored to make it suitable for a summative criterion, as in the example of checking the quality of medical summaries in the record (*see* below).

For difficult-to-measure criteria, a formative criterion may provide a better method of measurement. Clinicians should listen to patients. Measuring and judging whether this had occurred to the satisfaction of a professional colleague or a patient would vary. Therefore discussion of the principles and video of consultations would help this. If a grading system were developed this could be used to assess the clinicians' ability to listen to patients. There are difficulties with this approach and the measurement tool has to be well targeted. One would have to ensure that the assessment tool was measuring listening skills and not the ability to make a video.

Some clinical actions are likely to be too difficult to measure in a sufficiently robust and efficient way for use in a scheme. Therefore some clinical areas remain without measurements; for example, the therapeutic relationship between the doctor and the patient in depression. There are many scales and the area is important but there is no accurate reliable method that could be used within reasonable resource constraints.

Setting standards

The standard is the level of achievement expected for each individual criterion. Some criteria are difficult to achieve, others less so. If a parameter is to be both measured and controlled, the proportion measured is likely to be higher than the proportion controlled. The setting of standards implies a summative criterion. There is no necessity to decide standards before the assessment for formative criteria. The evidence can be assessed at the visit but it is difficult to fail a formative criterion if there is no summative element. This is dealt with by the formulation of the criterion; either no specific standard is required or improvement can be specified.

Review of the evidence suggests that process measures, say the measurement of blood pressure or cholesterol, can be achieved in 80% of populations in most cases. The very best have achieved 95% measurement of criteria.[33,34] This is without exclusions for patient choice. A higher level should be possible if patients can be excluded for reasons of choice or clinical exceptions. Similarly some patients have to be excluded for clinical reasons. If the proportion likely to be excluded for clinical reasons is high then it is usually better not to use the criterion.

Very high standards can be achieved in single areas but the cost is high in effort and time. It is possible that high levels of achievement in one area may detract from achievement across multiple areas. Challenging standards below the maximum achievable in individual areas can be set using the same percentage for most areas, with variation if there are special reasons.

For outcomes, setting standards is more difficult. Each area is individual and experience and judgement are required. Ultimately it is the implementation of change and review of the standards that can be achieved that decides levels for the future.

If there are likely to be high levels of measurement of a parameter but the clinical situation is complicated, only a small proportion can be controlled and measured. In this situation it is better to avoid a summative criterion and standard for the area. If it is necessary to measure the parameter, a formative criterion or indirect measurement of the area by a different method may be more suitable.

Decide on a data collection method

After criteria have been set it is necessary to establish a method to decide if the criteria and its standard have been met. The evidence can come in many formats. Depending on the nature of the criteria, this could be written evidence, a computer printout, the production of a statement from a third party or a visit to the practice for a detailed review of the evidence of attainment. Most current schemes (Fellowship by Assessment, Quality Practice Award, PRICCE) require a mix of methods and a practice visit. A visit is usual because some criteria require sight of the notes or the practice environment. Observing how a practice works and speaking to those who work there can reveal a lot.

Data collection can take a great deal of time and effort. If the data are already recorded in a known way on a computer database they can be audited by a computer search. Alternatively individual audits of the computer database can be collated and used as a summary of performance. More effort is required to access notes and check for a measurement to perform a manual audit. If this is to be done the size of the sample to be measured has to be specified. Formative criteria require the production of work for discussion. This has to be created and sometimes requires to be audited, improved and a second audit performed to complete the cycle. For each criterion it is necessary to have a data collection method and a format in which to present the data.

Develop this or design another system to facilitate data collection

If the aim is to use a computer system to perform a previously programmed search and produce a standardised report, the data have to be in a useable format. Some of the requirements sound obvious but the internal architecture of computer systems varies. Computer systems can only measure the data recorded on them. The criteria need to be worded to take this into account and they need to allow data entry in a simple and reliable way. Once the data are entered, the computer has to treat them as a single data set. Different computer software systems record data in different ways. This can affect the apparent achievement of criteria and standards. There are many issues to address when producing reports that mean the same thing from several different computer systems.

The clinician has to record all the data for the same illness in the same place, usually under the Read code for the illness. There need to be codes for all the data to be collected. If a criterion requires that something is not present or should be normal then there needs to be a Read code for that situation. If exclusions are to be allowed for patient choice or clinical contraindications to treatment then there needs to be a Read code for that or the system cannot include them. For example, aspirin is a good idea for most patients after myocardial infarction (MI) but should not be given if the patient has had a duodenal ulcer. A Read code for medically contraindicated situations is required, preferably with a reason. Specific Read codes can be created to allow particular data to be recorded.

Design a reporting and assessment system

Once the nature of the data to be collected and the format in which they are to be collected are known, a system is required to review the figures and verify whether they are correct. This is then used to decide whether success has been achieved and, if appropriate, makes awards or payment. This could be collecting computer printouts, which are known to reflect the computer database, or it could mean review of written data and a visit to the practice to confirm what has been achieved. In a formative process some form of contact and review is required.

There is the option of using a computer report alone. If there are criteria that require review in the clinical unit there is the option of asking for detailed written work in advance or actually looking for something on a visit.

Box 6.8   Methods for assessing criteria

For example, a criterion might say:

'The practice will have a policy for transferring telephone calls to the out-of-hours provider.'

This could be met by asking for a written policy including a lot of detail, the message used and who will switch the phone over.

Alternatively, a receptionist could demonstrate the method in two minutes on a visit to the practice.

There is a balance between asking for everything in writing and checking on the day. Checking on the day reduces paperwork but it will lead to more misunderstandings and occasionally finding that internal systems are not adequate.

Some criteria require checking within the practice; for example, 'the records will be legible and contain sufficient information for the next consultation'. This will require review of a number of records and a judgement.

A data-gathering visit functions as a fixed point on the assessment timescale. The practice has to achieve by a date and the assessors have to review the evidence by that date. It allows the assessors to look at the criteria that cannot be measured by pre-prepared material. The factual accuracy of the data can be checked by looking at the source of the data.

The visit also allows for many other issues to be discussed. The practice could be congratulated on achievement. Steady improvement and, at the higher levels, the retention of previously achieved levels of care are difficult. If the criteria and standards are challenging then achievement merits recognition. Other issues noted at another time or during the visit could be raised. These could be soft, formative thoughts and impressions or specific issues. Future developments could be discussed. Advice or specific suggestions from the assessors can be helpful when considering a new task, particularly if the assessors are also managers and use their access to the resources required for that development.

The values and objectives of the assessors could also be discussed. This is likely to be a developmental process for all concerned.

Any scheme runs the risk of the assessors getting it wrong on the day. This can be reduced by clarity about what is required so the practice will know, when it is producing the data, whether it has met the criteria or not. The more judgement that is required on the day, the more there is potential for not achieving a uniform assessment technique. Well-specified summative criteria with data produced by a standard method before the visit are least likely to result in appeals.

Train assessors

A scheme requires sufficient assessors. They need to be appropriately skilled and able to accomplish the tasks expected of them. This in part relates to their main job role and their ability. It is also related to their ability to do the assessments in a uniform way. The training would initially concentrate on the meaning of the criteria and standards and the supporting guidance in order to produce a uniform approach. A training programme should describe the standards and exactly what is expected and the skills of visiting a practice and helping colleagues with change. This requires a working knowledge of the issues faced by the unit being assessed. Once the issues have been exposed there is a need for practical skills and ideas to help development and guide rather than push participants towards solutions. This reflects the attitudes of the assessors. There is a need to explore the assessors' attitudes to and methods of change management. They will need to understand managing a practice as well as the members of the practice do. They will need to understand how to improve a practice in practical ways for the areas covered by criteria. Their teaching skills and the ability to solve practical problems that inevitably arise are important.

Visits to practices can also uncover poor organisations that are not developing. It is expected that the majority of clinical units will strive to improve clinical care and that providing resources will produce improvement. If the unit starts from a low level then improvement is just as valuable but the highest standards will take time to achieve. Assisting these units is likely to be challenging, as the assessors may not have the knowledge and skills to start at the base of practice development. However, all current practices developed from much smaller, less developed units in a stepwise fashion. The facilities and skills to start with a basic clinical unit and help it improve need to be available to the assessment team.

If extremely poor or dangerous practice is discovered it will require immediate action. The action depends on whether the deficiency is in clinical skills or the management of the organisation. Clinical skills of individuals are referred to professional organisations, for example the GMC or NMC. Management deficiencies can be improved by appointing more staff and specific help.

Once assessors are working there is a need for a further system to review the performance of the assessors. Uniform assessment is difficult and costly to achieve.

Who should be on the visiting team?

This is determined by the nature of the assessment process to be used and the sensitivity of the data to be looked at. For a formative assessment there is a necessity for a detailed discussion of the evidence produced. A professional from the same peer group is required. This could be a clinician for clinical issues but may be a manager for other members of the team. If the assessment is summative and there is an amount of preparation, the visit does not require peers to assess the data. If clinical data are to be observed clinicians should perform that part of the assessment. Detailed discussion of subsequent developments will require a high-level manager with an understanding of local resource allocation policy and the ability to make decisions.

Worked example for the process of creating criteria and standards

It is easier to understand the reasons and purpose of the decisions that go into creating a criterion and standard through a worked example. Two areas of importance in general practice that lead to different kinds of criteria are the control of hypertension and the creation of summaries. The development of each set of criteria will be considered in turn.

Hypertension

Hypertension is important because of the substantial premature morbidity and mortality occurring if it goes untreated. The initial thoughts about hypertension are that it should be monitored and the reading recorded and that it should be controlled. This represents two different actions and therefore two criteria and a register will be required. There is evidence that blood pressure is not currently controlled and that improving it will improve the health of patients and therefore clinicians are likely to accept a criterion in this area. Monitoring and treatment of hypertension are under the direct control of GP practices. Data on blood pressures are currently collected although they are probably not complete. Some of the recording is on computer and some on paper, with minimal overlap, leading to two different data sets.

Measurement of blood pressure and control is amenable to a summative assessment method. The proportion measured and the proportion controlled could be compared with the total population of hypertensive patients in the practice. In order to do this, a definition of hypertension and a review period have to be selected. A formative criterion could also be developed; for example, a practice will produce a written policy for management of hypertension and audit care for one audit cycle and show improvement. The practice would be expected to review the evidence and produce a policy, which would be used by the practice. This would require detailed study of the evidence and discussion of the results. The audit would be produced and show improvement. This would result in detailed discussion with the assessors. There is no requirement to reach a specific level but improvement in management is required. In order to improve care to defined levels and produce a uniform assessment, a summative assessment seems appropriate.

Review of the evidence base suggests that the current requirement for blood pressure control is below 140/85. This is likely to be difficult to achieve in most patients without inducing hypotension in some. Therefore an audit criterion or indicator is required. The criterion now becomes an indicator requiring control of blood pressure to 150/90 or below.

It could be measured by sampling a fixed number of records on the disease register both for the proportion of hypertensive patients with a recorded blood pressure and for the last reading. An average of several readings could be taken but this would make it difficult to improve care in the recording period. The alternative would be to enter the readings into a computer database and perform a search of the complete database. Once the data are entered this requires less time and provides better data.

The degree to which a practice can measure and control blood pressure is a guess based on experience. The practices in the PRICCE scheme achieved 100% measurement and 85% control for recording within one year. Exclusions were required to get to this level. A lower level seems appropriate for general introduction – say 90% measurement and 70% control. Any standards set have to be left for review if too easy or too difficult.

As a computer audit is the preferred measurement option it remains to choose a standard Read code for hypertension, design the system to collect the numeric value of a blood pressure and design a computer audit to produce figures on a set date. The data and search method is unlikely to be improved on by inspecting the notes. If the notes showed different levels to the computer it would raise suspicions but checking the computer data would reveal the same figures.

Table 6.2 Development of example criteria for hypertension.

Area to review	Hypertension
Why is it important?	Control of hypertension will reduce morbidity and mortality
Suggested criteria	Presence of a disease register for hypertensive patients Blood pressure is measured in hypertensive patients Blood pressure is controlled in hypertensive patients
Will achieving the criteria improve care?	Yes
Can it be changed by the practice?	Yes
Are data already collected?	Yes (could be on computer or in paper records)
Measurement method	Summative
Refined criteria after deciding formative or summative measurement method	Blood pressure will be recorded in hypertensive patients Recorded blood pressure will be below (say) 160/90 within the last 12 months
Refined criteria after comparison with evidence and national guidance	Blood pressure will be recorded in hypertensive patients Blood pressure will be below 140/85 within the last six months
Moderate to increase the population to be measured (create indicator)	Blood pressure will be recorded in hypertensive patients Blood pressure will be 150/90 or below within the last nine months
Measurement method	Choice of audit of (say) 200 hypertensive patients' records or computer audit of last BP in all hypertensive patients Manual record of last recorded blood pressure for (say) 200 patients Computer search of all hypertensive patients' last blood pressure
Set standard	Measurement level 90% Control level 70%
IT system changes	If the practice enters the data, computer audit of whole population possible. Development of a standard audit tool for computer system
Reporting system	Computer printout of situation on a particular date

Summaries

Up-to-date summaries of care are important and recommended in *Good Medical Practice for GPs*. The summary has to be fit for purpose and that will vary depending on how it is displayed. The summary should contain important data without confusing the reader with unnecessary information. Computers give the option of selecting data. Paper records cannot be filtered and the policy may vary for a paper or computer summary. Summaries are important because the clinician benefits from knowing what has happened in the past. Accurate records can also be used to find patients with the same diagnosis to deliver care proactively to them. Summaries also allow the development of disease registers which need to be available for the practice and not necessarily the individual clinician. This is fundamental to delivering chronic disease management. The presence and accuracy of summaries are in the control of the practice.

As the format of summaries will vary because of local circumstances, it is difficult to define what should be in a summary. If the detail is described, the practice has little or no autonomy and damage could be done if the enforced ideas are perceived to damage care. A formative criterion that requires the practice to create a method to generate summaries will get around this difficulty. However, there is not a uniform approach and variable outcomes could occur. Alternatively, the reason for creating summaries could be used to create a summative criterion that achieves something similar. When summaries are created or checked, the drug index is useful because there has to be a reason for drug prescribing and it can be used as a way of selecting which patients to look for or a particular diagnosis. In reality this was a significant method used in the creation of summaries in the first place. It follows that each illness serious enough to require a repeat medication should be recorded in the summary. This would record most illnesses but some, like operations and cured cancers, do not require long-term medication. It is also possible to specify that certain illnesses should be recorded on a disease index. The presence of these diseases on a drug index then becomes a reason for an entry in the summary. This documentation, whilst not completely comprehensive, can be formulated into a summative criterion. Both options are shown in the example as they measure different things.

A formative criterion is not much changed by consulting the evidence. That is for the practice to do in writing its internal policy. There is no national evidence for which drugs should have an attached diagnosis or which disease registers are helpful. There is also no need to change the criterion to create an indicator. It has not been standard practice to record indications for repeat medications. Therefore a prospective indicator is appropriate to allow new diagnoses to be entered as new drugs are started.

Both criteria are difficult to measure. Checking whether the summary accurately reflects the records is a time-consuming task that requires the skills of a clinician. Therefore a number of records, usually small, are sampled to assess whether the criterion is met for each individual set of notes. A check for the accuracy of a disease register would require a similar review of records. A review of whether there was a summary entry appropriate for each repeat medication can be accomplished without a notes search but still requires a clinician. It would be possible to create a formal link between each drug and an indication within a computer system. In time this would provide the ability to perform a computer search of the whole practice population. This would be useful for assessment and for the practice trying to improve the database and quality of its records.

The standard required for notes summaries has to be high in order for the records to be reliable. If a low proportion are summarised the doctor has to check if anything is missing each time. A significant proportion of practice records, particularly of children, include no serious illnesses and do not require any summary entries. The creation and checking of summaries take a long

Table 6.3 Development of example criteria for summaries of the medical record.

Area to review	Summaries	
Why is it important?	Having the major illnesses known to the clinician aids diagnosis and treatment. It needs to be comprehensive to show the important diagnoses and small enough to use on the available display mechanism Patients with specific diseases can be found to target care	
Suggested criteria	Summaries are available in the consultation Disease registers are available in the practice	
Will achieving the criteria improve care?	Yes, if the summaries and disease registers are used	
Can it be changed by the practice?	Yes	
Are data already collected?	Yes (could be on computer or in paper records)	
Measurement method	Formative	Summative
Refined criteria after deciding formative or summative measurement method	The practice will produce a protocol for writing summaries Summaries will be available in clinical records	A clinical indication will be available in the record summary for each repeat medication A disease register will be available for all patients with (say) hypertension
Refined criteria after comparison with evidence and national guidance	The practice will produce a protocol for writing summaries Summaries will be available in clinical records	A clinical indication will be available in the record summary for each repeat medication A disease register will be available for all patients with (say) hypertension
Moderate to increase the population to be measured (create indicator)	The practice will produce a protocol for writing summaries Summaries will be available in clinical records	A clinical indication will be available in the record summary for each repeat medication for all new diagnoses after 1.4.2004 A disease register will be available for all patients with (say) hypertension
Measurement method	Review practice summary protocol. Review (say) 20 records to see if summaries accurate by reviewing clinical data	Review of notes or computer entry for (say) 20 records to see if there is an indication for each drug Or create checkable computer link between repeat medication and indication then computer search of all repeat medication Audit of patients on hypertensive medications to see if high blood pressures recorded and whether hypertension marker recorded
Set standard	Set two levels for the percentage of accurate summaries to allow for an increase over time: 60% and 80%	80%
IT system changes	Not amenable to computer audit	Requires the development of a link between repeat medicines and the indication Development of a standard audit tool for computer system
Reporting system	Visit to the practice to review the policy and inspect notes	Visit to the practice to review the policy and inspect notes After change to IT system, computer printout of situation on a particular date

time and a great deal of work. Multiple standards will reward partial achievement of summarisation.

No change to the IT system will facilitate assessment of the level of summarisation for the manual method used initially. Changes to the system could change the display method and amount of data collected. Linking drugs and indications would have a large impact on this criterion.

Constraints on setting criteria

Whilst many interventions have been shown to benefit patients in clinical trials, few have been large enough to review the intervention when implemented across a whole local population. Clinical trials exclude patients with multiple illnesses and multiple drug interactions. They are therefore a useful pointer for general practice but only apply to specific subgroups. Relatively little chronic disease management has been implemented universally across general practice.[4] Evidence is often not available to show the effectiveness of specific interventions when implemented in a GP population. It is therefore necessary to select diseases in clinical areas where the evidence is strong. There is also a limit to the number of criteria that can be measured because of the additional work of monitoring itself. This is particularly so if preparation and formative assessment is required.

The amount of evidence available for improvement in population health by implementing specific interventions is limited so only a few diseases can be specified by this method. Even in these areas, the number of criteria that have validity across the population is limited.

These include:

- Angina
- Post MI
- Other vascular disease: cerebrovascular accident (CVA), transient ischaemic attacks (TIA), peripheral vascular disease
- Left ventricular dysfunction
- Chronic obstructive pulmonary disease (COPD)
- Hypothyroidism
- Diabetes
- Some asthma criteria.

There are no references to check against this list. It represents the common illnesses where work has been performed in general practice and where control can in some way be measured by numbers. It is to be hoped that in time it will become the norm to trial particular interventions in disease in a population setting where there is co-morbidity, multiple medication and patient choice that make implementation of clinical trial results for populations difficult.

Preparatory work

Schemes assume a minimum standard of ability and infrastructure among participating units. Practices below this minimum level may not be able to use the scheme if their starting point is well below other scheme participants. At some level there has to be the capacity to develop within a scheme. As a minimum this has to be the existing statutory requirement. There have to be some buildings and staff to work with and the participants need to be able to create and use educational tools. In many schemes inclusion criteria are set and only those practices that meet the criteria can enter. This gives a uniform improvement requirement and the scheme and education and training are geared to this.

Participants will need to be persuaded that entering the scheme is beneficial by the publicity for the scheme. PCO managers need to have the ability to obtain the infrastructure required by the scheme. They also need to put in place the assessment methodology.

Part 2

How the contract was created

Chapter 7

Features of the 2003 General Medical Services (GMS) contract

The 2003 GMS contract is a contract between the PCO and the practice as an organisation. The practice agrees to provide specified services in return for specified resources. There is no longer a contract with individual doctors. This allows other clinicians or managers to make and manage the contract, on their own or as partners of the GPs. Some or all of the doctors can be salaried by the practice. Contract specifications for salaried doctors have been produced to be used as minimum specifications.

Practices can opt out of care for patients between 6.30 p.m. and 8 a.m. They can provide the services themselves or ask the PCO to provide them.

In order to allow practices to control their workload if they have difficulty finding staff, the categories of essential services, additional services and enhanced services have been created. All practices have to provide essential services, defined as services to patients who are or believe themselves to be ill. Additional services will be provided by most practices but, with agreement, the practice can ask the PCO to provide them. The Quality and Outcomes Framework (see Ch. 8) specifies how quality will be measured in essential and additional services.

Practices have the option of providing enhanced services, some of which are specified nationally (directed national enhanced services and national enhanced services) and others locally (locally enhanced services). Enhanced services are outside the Quality and Outcomes Framework.

The PCO is required to deliver these standards for its population whether the practices deliver the services or not. This is called the patient guarantee. Practices are preferred bidders for some services (essential services, additional services and directed enhanced services) and, if they provide them, they are guaranteed the necessary resources. The PCO has the option of contracting with practices or other organisations for the remaining services (national enhanced services, local enhanced services). If practices do not meet the access targets the PCO will retain the resources to spend on alternative services to achieve access. In most instances the PCO will also be contracting for the out-of-hours service. PCOs can directly employ doctors and practice staff.

The provision of resources for practice premises and information technology becomes the responsibility of the PCO. New flexibilities are available for premises: the PCO can buy land for practices to use when a rapid decision is required and land is in demand. Practices will have the option of increasing rents on a notional rental basis or annual inflation uplifts. PCOs will be able to take over the lease between a practice and its landlord as a tenant of last resort, to maintain the availability of premises for the NHS. PCOs will fully fund practice IT systems and assist with future development and integration into NHS information technology.

New training opportunities and a career structure will be available to GPs. There is the option of spending time learning new clinical skills, special interest development and clinical leadership. The funding is available to enable practices to release GPs for this work. Practices also have the funds to enable staff to attend training and development with reduced commitment. The protected learning time required for professional development and regular education and time for personal appraisal is also funded through the global sum.

The payment structure for practices is described. The largest element is the global sum, which is proportionate to the number of patients registered with the practice. This is multiplied by a factor representing the difficulty and workload involved in looking after the particular case mix. This will create a notional list. The payments for quality and enhanced services are added to this. Additional personal seniority payments will be available for GMS doctors but not salaried doctors. Maternity and sickness benefits will be provided with payments from the PCO. The networks of payments for individual services available under the old GMS contract are no longer available.

Practices have flexibility to manage themselves and employ different grades of staff to provide services that satisfy quality outcome measures.

The quality required for the contract is specified in several places. The contractual and statutory requirements apply to all practices while the Quality and Outcomes Framework is voluntary but releases considerable funds to practices. A practice that decided not to enter the framework would struggle for income. Patient access criteria are specified in the Quality and Outcomes Framework and the quality requirements of the enhanced services are individually specified.

The net effect is to substantially increase the resources and incomes available to GPs. The pay rates of salaried doctors, nurses and staff are unchanged but affected by the general increase in incomes occurring for NHS staff.

Quality in the 2003 GMS contract

The requests of government and the GP negotiators on behalf of GPs have been set out earlier. The initial negotiations resulted in the production of a framework and principles for the new GMS contract that were agreed with the four UK governments and accepted by the GPs in a ballot.[40]

This described payments to practices for achieving quality, organised as a scheme with direct payment for achieving clinical and organisational criteria and for consulting on the patient perspective. It described increasing levels of achievement for progressively increasing numbers of criteria and higher standards. Exception reporting was to be allowed for clinical contraindications to treatment. A high trust reporting system was promised with minimal extra bureaucracy and a standard nationally agreed format. A visit to the practice by PCO representatives to validate performance was included.

The Quality and Outcomes Framework was developed to fulfil this requirement.[41] This describes how quality will be measured and paid for in the 2003 GMS contract. Previous experience of contracts and change management schemes was used to create a series of criteria. Clinical and organisational criteria and standards were developed using the principles described earlier. For each criterion, a method of measurement was decided which is to be reviewed on a visit to the practice. The reason for the choice of each area included, the choice of the indicator itself, the measurement method and the preferred Read code are listed in the supporting guidance.[41]

The payment structure was also described to allow the framework to be used for financial allocations to practices. The formulas were subject to review and the agreed documentation further interpreted after publication. The Quality and Outcomes Framework and the principles have remained unchanged.

The contract documentation also describes the structure available for individuals to undertake training outside the practice for clinical and organisational leadership in the NHS.

What is special about writing a scheme as a national government contract?

A contract is more than a quality scheme. There is little ability to obtain primary medical care outside the NHS and therefore an NHS contract has to provide for all patients and be appropriate for all GPs and staff. It has to work from multiple entry points for practices with different degrees of organisation and not leave out any groups. It has to work for practices with few resources, struggling to cope and offering little chronic disease management, as well as well-developed practices offering high-quality services. It has to be fair and open to appeal. It has to consider the minimum acceptable standard and provide methods for improvement from every level. It has to improve all practices to a single, uniformly high level by reducing variation between practices, without harming development of the best.

The criteria chosen have to be acceptable to all stakeholders, clinicians, governments, managers and patients.

The resources available to practices as they improve quality should reflect the additional work and cost involved in that development. The income payment remaining for the partners after expenses should rank the achievement of the practice and reflect the work and ability required. The measurement system should reflect this need and intrude as little as possible on clinical time with patients. Appeals should be available but the design of the measurement system should minimise the disagreements and need for appeals by its clarity.

Individuals working within the NHS have to be treated fairly and the government has a duty of care to those employed within the system. In previous general practice contracts there was no mechanism to monitor the terms and conditions of service of staff. An NHS contract should specify how protection of employees is to be achieved by detailing the provision of contracts, training and appraisal.

Training and development of individuals are expensive and practices have to decide whether some forms of training are cost effective. Movement between practices and dissemination of ideas or the creation of local leaders are of benefit to the NHS as a whole. An NHS scheme should balance this conflict and provide mechanisms to promote skills development. Resources should be available for individuals to develop their skills as part of practice improvement. In addition, opportunities and funding to develop other skills in addition to practice experience are required.

The NHS is required to demonstrate that high-quality care is being provided for all. Clinical quality and audited standards of care should be provided for whole populations of patients. The NHS requires the collection of data to demonstrate its performance.

The NHS funds and controls the environment in which GP practices operate. This provides the opportunity to change the funding and resources available in the rest of the health service. The contract does not include primary care outside the practice because it has a different management structure. Other primary care facilities, funding for medicines and secondary care provision can be changed to meet the implications for workload elsewhere implicit in improved quality in general practice.

The quality improvement requested and the assessment system should complement the measurement methods used for PCO managers. CHI does not inspect practices but the contract requirements should broadly align with the requirements of the PCO inspection and other government priorities for the PCO.

Chapter 8

The Quality and Outcomes Framework

The Quality and Outcomes Framework is voluntary and practices can decide whether to enter and which level they wish to achieve. Payments are linked to achievement of the individual criteria and standards. Each criterion has a number of points allocated to it. The number of points varies according to the amount and difficulty of the work required to achieve success with each criterion. In addition, contractual and statutory requirements have been published which specify minimum standards, which are not voluntary, and no payments attach to these.

The whole document is called a framework. It is organised into four domains: clinical, organisational, patient experience and additional services. Each domain is divided into a number of areas. Each area is subdivided into individual indicators (audit criteria).

Table 8.1   The structure of the Quality and Outcomes Framework.

Domain	Clinical	Organisational	Patient experience	Additional services
Area	Ten clinical areas	Five organisational areas	Two areas	Four clinical areas that practices can choose to be involved with to a specified standard

Most of the criteria are summative and standards have been set. Computer data can be used for most clinical and some organisational criteria. In this way high trust monitoring can be created with the production of a computer-based report for much of the data required for the assessment. For the remaining criteria, the information to be produced is clear and practices can be confident of their performance before the visit.

Supporting documentation gives the reason why the area was chosen, the evidence for choosing the individual criteria and the rationale for the individual indicators (audit criteria).[41] The data collection and assessment method is described.

The four domains

Clinical domain

The clinical domain is constructed using clinical criteria and standards in 10 areas.

- Coronary heart disease (CHD) including left ventricular dysfunction (LVD)
- Stroke and TIA
- Hypertension
- Hypothyroidism
- Diabetes
- Mental health
- COPD
- Asthma
- Epilepsy
- Cancer.

The criteria are summative and the vast majority of the data can all be collected from the computer system. This will produce a uniform measurement method, clarity and accurate ranking between practices of outcomes without specifying process. As a result of the data collection, the NHS will know the incidence of these diseases and the level of control across the whole population. Any improvements in care due to the efforts of practices will also be known. The collection of summative data allows autonomy of method.

There is a requirement to create an accurate register for the disease in question. The indicators for each clinical area are described and for each there is a standard. This represents the upper level for which payments will be available. For the criteria that specify process measures, for example the measurement of blood pressure, a common standard of 90% achievement has been selected. For the outcome measures, for example control of blood pressure to below 150/90, standards have been individually set. It is accepted that practices can only request patients to make changes. Patients should be informed and able to make that choice. If the patient refuses to have treatment they can be excluded from the population for that particular criterion. For individual criteria there may be other specific exclusions mentioned in the guidance or agreed at the time of the assessment visit. It is believed that for all criteria the standards can be reached without describing exclusions. Therefore if the practice has achieved the levels there is no need to discuss exclusions but the option remains if there are good reasons.

Principles of the clinical domain

- Accurate and complete disease register
- Measure the criterion
- Upper and lower level standards for each criterion
- Measure control of the disease
- Variable maximum control levels for each criterion
- Exclusion of patients for patient choice and clinical reasons

---

Organisational domain

The organisational criteria are designed to achieve two functions. First, they list tasks that are required to prove compliance with legislation or good practice. Second, they signpost the organisational tasks required to improve a practice.

Practices vary enormously in situation, patients and current capability. The domains are designed to start with a basic minimum requirement and build to a complex practice. The organisational domain mirrors the increasingly complex systems that are required to take a practice from disease-orientated, reactive medicine with GPs and few staff to a complex organisation with many professionals. Each professional has a role and others rely on that role being accomplished. This has to continue even if individuals are absent or move on to new jobs. A large practice would expect to proactively manage chronic disease as well as the immediate needs of patients. At the highest levels this organisation will be capable of understanding how it performs its task and developing new research and systems to improve clinical and organisational management – a learning organisation. The framework is designed to help practice and PCO personnel focus on important areas of practice development. The areas covered are the same as for clinical governance. However, clinical governance requires the checking and implementing of specific processes. The organisational domain specifies the outcomes practices are expected to achieve without specifying the method.

The criteria are designed to be measurable in a reproducible way across the country to equalise standards. Some require the creation of policies or written material and therefore have a formative element. For each criterion there is a description of how the practice will meet it and the evidence that is to be presented to the PCO to demonstrate that the criterion has been achieved. The criteria themselves and the accompanying guidance have been written to minimise the amount of preparatory time required. As far as possible, if a policy is required the assessors will not need to see it before the visit but will expect to see one on the day. Speaking to the staff at the visit will give further evidence of the use of practice-developed systems. In this way many items can be dealt with speedily and efficiently. In the event of disagreements the criteria, standards and evidence required are clear.

The organisational standards have been subdivided in several ways. The Quality and Outcomes Framework is voluntary but there are a number of criteria that are important and based on legal requirements. They are not thought to be universally implemented or subject to change and the criteria specify what practices are expected to produce to verify compliance. Therefore practices and PCOs can be confident they are achieved. It is not expected that they will be checked in detail on every visit. The standard expected for implementation of the contractual and statutory requirements is 100%.

Some criteria measure an important parameter, others act as examples of the ability to perform a task or demonstrate that a system works. For example, the contract measures the expiry dates of some drugs but all drugs need to be up to date. The measured item is intended to show the presence of an effective system, which can be used in other areas or in this case for other drugs.

The criteria are divided into five areas. Each criterion is separately scored for points. This allows practices to develop at different speeds with different domains yet reduce the complexity of the payment system. The five domains are:

- Records and information about patients
- Communicating with patients
- Education and training
- Practice management
- Medicines management.

Principles of the organisational framework

- Criteria are developmental
- Minimum level of existing statutes for all practices
- Measurable in a simple and reliable way
- Points (and resources) allocated in proportion to the difficulty of the task
- Some criteria function as markers that generic skills are present in the practice
- Those skills should be used to improve the rest of the practice's work
- Success with the criteria achieves clinical governance requirements

---

The framework is not divided into groups of criteria or levels and practices can choose which criteria they wish to achieve. The criteria conform to increasing sophistication from a base level practice that has few staff and facilities through improving to the steady-state practices that have already achieved quality and need to maintain that high level of achievement. Most practices should already be achieving some of the criteria but only a relatively small number are likely to be achieving all of them.

Patient experience

The patient experience domain is intended to provide information on how the patients view the practice. With three individual pieces of work, the practice can consult and meet patient needs. A choice of tools has been agreed and others could be added later.

Patient questionnaires

Two patient questionnaires (the General Practice Assessment Questionnaire – GPAQ – and the Improving Practices Questionnaire – IPQ*) have been accepted as valid measures of patient views, to be issued to patients on an annual basis. They can be posted or given out in the surgery. Patients have

---

* GPAQ is available at www.gpaq.info
IPQ is available at latis.ex.uk/cfep/ipq.htm

been asked for their views of practices many times and the result is usually very positive. The questionnaires aim to look at the experience of the practice not measured by the clinical and organisational standards. They look at access, the quality of the consultation itself and the information given out, the quality of the premises and the views of other parts of the practice the patients have experienced.

The questionnaires are standardised and have been used extensively in British general practice so it is possible to compare practice and personal performance with experience elsewhere in the United Kingdom. The GPAQ instrument is free to use and printed copies can be obtained for a fee. The IPQ instrument is not available free but the cost includes printed questionnaires and analysis.

The three areas of the contract require a questionnaire to be used initially, for a report and inferences to be taken and actioned and for the practice to discuss the anonymous results with a third party representing either patients or the PCO. In this way the views of patients are fed to the practice, which is expected to use the results to make its services more appropriate for local patients. Practices are not marked according to the absolute values of the results and patient views do not affect income. This criterion is formative and reviewed by either patient representatives from the practice or a non-executive director of the PCO.

It has been done this way to encourage practices to talk to their patients and configure services to meet their needs. The existing satisfaction levels of practice do not suggest there is a problem and local fine-tuning is likely to be the outcome of the consultation exercise.

Appointment length

The contract rewards the use of 10-minute appointments for routine consultations. Evidence shows that patients value longer consultation times. The intention is for more issues to be completed in one consultation but this is difficult to measure directly. The individual parts of the consultation, history, prescribing and explanation are reviewed in the questionnaires but length of consultations in general practice itself equates with improved outcomes.[42] Ten minutes is specified because the current evidence relates to that figure.

Consulting with patients about other issues

The contract does not require other consultations about experience but, as practices become used to the concept of consulting patients, refinements may be introduced in addition to or in place of the two named questionnaires.

Principles required in the patient experience

- Consultation with patients by questionnaire
- Acting on results
- Practices not ranked by the values obtained
- Aim is to inform practices of their own patients' requests
- Rewards 10-minute appointments

Additional medical services

As practices can opt out of some services, not all practices will provide additional medical services. A similar process has been used for these areas to create a list of organisational criteria. Each is a separate free-standing entity. The areas covered are:

* Cervical screening
* Child health surveillance
* Maternity services
* Contraceptive services.

Most of the criteria require the creation of or adherence to local policies. Only one, cervical cytology, is summative and has a standard. All are areas that attracted separate payments under the old GMS contract. There is no gradation for partial achievement, except in cervical cytology, and points are awarded for agreeing to provide the service. If practices choose not to provide these services the PCO can provide or purchase them elsewhere to the same criteria. In many cases the requirements for following up smear defaulters will be provided centrally by the PCO.

Payments

The four domains

As described earlier, each criterion has a number of points attached which give relative weightings to the achievement of each criterion. For each summative criterion in the clinical domain, an upper standard has been set. The lowest level of achievement attracting payment is 25% for any criterion. The points are calculated to be the proportion of the difference between the lower standard and the upper standard multiplied by the points available for that criterion. The lower standard is always 25%.

Box 8.1 Working out the points achieved from the percentage with controlled disease in the clinical domain

For example, in hypertension, a criterion reads: 'The percentage of patients with hypertension in whom the last blood pressure (measured in the last nine months) is 150/90 or less'. The points are 56 and the upper standard (maximum threshold) is 70%. If the practice has achieved this criterion in 55% of patients they would receive $(55-25)/(70-25) \times 56$ points or $30/45 \times 56$ points or 37.33 points.

Once the practice has achieved the upper threshold the maximum number of points is achieved and further improvement does not attract further payment.

In the organisational and patient experience domains each criterion has a points value which is achieved if the criterion is met in full; there is no gradation for partial achievement. In additional services one criterion, cervical cytology, has a graded criterion to calculate the points achieved but all the others relate to meeting the criterion in its entirety.

Achievement of the contractual and statutory requirements is expected of all practices. There is no payment for achieving them. If deficiencies are found, practices are not meeting professional codes of conduct or breaching the law, they are expected to remedy the problem.

Holistic care payments

Patients want to be treated well for all their illnesses and do not want the professionals treating them to ignore whole illnesses or parts of illnesses. The practice has responsibility to produce systematic care across the range of illnesses inside and outside the contract. The difficulty with too much recording and setting criteria in certain areas is that it makes proof of total care impossible. However, breadth of care within the clinical domain has been encouraged by rewarding achievement across the clinical areas. The points score is calculated for all ten clinical areas. The eighth best score of the ten is taken as a proportion of the total points available for that clinical area. This proportion is multiplied by 100 to calculate a points score for the holistic care payment.

Box 8.2   Working out the points achieved in the holistic care payment

For example, the practice achieves 75% or more of the points available in seven of the ten clinical areas. It achieves 70% of the points in hypothyroidism (the eighth of ten clinical areas) and a lower proportion of the available points in the remaining two clinical areas. It would thus receive 70% of the 100 points available.

Quality practice payments

Similarly, performance across the four domains is rewarded by a separate payment in proportion to achievement in the third of four domains. There are 30 points available for quality practice payments.

Box 8.3   Working out the points achieved in the quality practice payment

For example, the points performance of the practice is:

- Clinical domain 60%
- Organisational domain 75%
- Patient perspective 100%
- Additional services 80%.

The third of four domains is the organisational domain and therefore 75% of 30 points (22.5 points) would be achieved for the quality practice payment.

Access payment

The ability to access the practice to allow patients to see a clinician is a requirement to deliver care. There is no evidence base to say how long that should be. In England *The NHS Plan* specifies the following target: 'By 2004, all patients will be able to see a primary care professional within 24 hours and a GP within 48 hours'. In Scotland *Our National Health: a plan for action, a plan for change* specifies 'access to an appropriate member of the primary healthcare team in 48 hours'. In Wales *The Future of Primary Care* specifies 'patients will be able to access an appropriate member of the primary care team within 24 hours of requesting an appointment and much sooner in an emergency'. The access target for Northern Ireland has yet to be released. The payment system allocates 50 points to the ability of patients to access the practice within the applicable national access target.

Using points to create payments

The points from the four domains add up to 1000 points. A further 50 points are available for the access payment. A monetary amount is attached to each payment, based on the average practice of 5500 patients and three GP principals. The payment to practices is proportionately adjusted for the notional number of patients to be treated. This is done using a formula which will be adjusted as information about disease prevalence is improved. In the first year of the contract, it will be £75, rising to £120 in the second year. A proportion of the payment (a third) would be available in advance in the preceding year as an aspiration payment to allow the practice to employ staff to achieve the quality standards. A reward payment (the full payment less the aspiration payment) would be released after the assessment visit when an accurate figure for points and money can be calculated.

The notional number of patients to be treated is related to the difficulty and workload expected to produce high-quality care. An initial formula (Carr-Hill) was used but will be subject to review as the factors influencing the difficulty of care and the numbers of patients to be treated in different settings become clear. If patients have not been recorded on disease registers there cannot be an accurate method for estimating the workload generated in practices by variable disease prevalence. The disease registers of the clinical domain will in time reveal the prevalence and influences on disease prevalence.

Contractual and statutory requirements

Twenty-five additional criteria from a range of organisational areas have been written to allow them to develop over time without changing the criteria themselves. The requirements will not change but the specific action required will evolve over time. For example, the obligation to provide contracts of employment to staff will not change but the form of the contract specified in legislation could change substantially.

Many are statutory obligations required by law. They are not comprehensive and do not describe every legal requirement. They are intended to guide practices and PCOs to areas that are likely to be important to general practice and specify how a practice can show it is meeting the legal requirements.

Other criteria are contractual requirements for the NHS, like the requirement to have a practice leaflet in a specific form.

Many of the criteria deal with the way staff are treated. There is now a clear statement that employment conditions and regular review (appraisal) are a requirement for an NHS general practice. The baseline requirements for records, confidentiality and data protection are also included. Information issued to patients about the practice is specified. There is a requirement to be non-discriminatory about which patients are taken on to the list. The practice list will now be open to all patients in the area of the practice or closed to all.

Maintenance of good practice in dealing with vaccines, recording batch numbers, contraindications and training and ability to deal with anaphylaxis is required. The recording of consent is required before certain specified procedures are carried out. If medicines and controlled drugs are stored, it must be in accordance with current legislation. Knowledge of child protection policies and a requirement to implement clinical governance are also included.

Practice attributes required for success with the Quality and Outcomes Framework

The Quality and Outcomes Framework requires many organisational abilities. As most of the criteria are summative, the development expected may not be the same as the criteria. The development and capabilities expected have been mapped across the criteria required for essential medical services. This includes the contractual and statutory criteria that are required of all practices and the three domains that all practices entering the Quality and Outcomes Framework are assessed against. The criteria for additional services have also been included.

The list is extensive and covers most aspects of a practice. These are the areas all practices will have to tackle to reach the top of the Quality and Outcomes Framework (*see* Table 8.2).

What is not included in the framework?

Many important areas of general practice are not amenable to the production of summative criteria. When care is related to the personality of the doctor or patient then individually tailored packages are produced by the doctor. Rules-based care, either in a protocol or an outcome-based summative criterion, will not measure success with the most important part of the job. Patient questionnaires provide some evidence but the patient may not know what else could have been available. Therefore discussion of individual cases and actions with colleagues provides an alternative route to measurement and improvement. The principal areas known to be left out at present are detailed in Table 8.3.

These issues could be tackled by formative criteria and peer review. Time would be required to produce criteria and standards for this. The specific areas described are mostly individual learning needs and not applicable to the practice as a whole. In time new schemes for individuals could be developed to help with these areas.

Table 8.2 How development needs and abilities are measured in the Quality and Outcomes Framework and contractual and statutory requirements.

Organisational area	Development need	Organisational standards*	Clinical standards	Patient questionnaire
Records and information about patients				
Disease registers	Presence of a record for case finding, audit education, changing treatment as medicine develops	Cross-collation of clinical diagnoses to repeat prescribing and review of summaries Legible records	Detailed scrutiny of a small number of registers	Not examined
Primary prevention	Case finding of illness	Smoking and hypertension	Review of incidence levels	Patient views of individual consultations
Secondary prevention	Case finding, updating data, data accuracy, change in clinical practice for individual patients	Presence of registers, 80% smear criteria Legible records	Achievement of outcome measures in several diseases	Not examined
Confidentiality	Holding data confidentially and informing patients about use	Caldecott guardian and the display of a notice	Not examined	Not examined
IT	Accurate disease registers and searchable database of specific parameters	Not included as this can be done without computer for individual illnesses	Databases must be present to produce data at higher contract levels	Not examined
Communicating with patients				
Opening hours and contact arrangements	Facilitating easy contact arrangements, appointment and telephone access	Description of contact arrangements and opening hours	Not measured	Specific questions on function
Relationships with patients	Respect and continuity, explanations, personal advice	Complaints system	Requires continuity and excellent relationships to persuade the patient to attend and re-attend for review	Directly questioned

Education and training

Administrative staff	Employment of appropriate grades, appropriate training Personal development planning Respect for colleagues' skills Functional teams	Contracts, appraisal, standard employment practices, specific job specifications	Achievement of criteria promotes respect for colleagues and development of complementary roles based on individual talents within a team	High-quality patient contact Skills to run the practice in a responsive way
Practice management staff	Employment of appropriate grades, appropriate training Personal development planning Respect for colleagues' skills Functional teams	Management change agenda to reach organisational framework requirements	Meeting learning needs to enable organisation or reorganisation of systems to achieve criteria and standards Review and change of methods when steady state reached	High-quality patient contact Skills to run the practice in a responsive way
Education of nurses	Employment of appropriate grades, appropriate training Personal development planning Respect for colleagues' skills Functional teams	Contracts, appraisal, standard employment practices, specific training on smears, checking of qualifications, staff job specifications	Achievement of criteria promotes respect for colleagues and development of complementary roles based on individual talents within a team	Clinical and communication skills
Education of doctors	Updating in the major disease areas, annual appraisal	Not examined	Doctors will often challenge clinical criteria, which leads to a review of evidence Will require development of skills to look at the evidence base	Clinical and communication skills

Table 8.2 Continued.

Organisational area	Development need	Organisational standards*	Clinical standards	Patient questionnaire
Practice management				
Practice policies	Locally appropriate methods of dealing with administrative tasks that work, are known to staff and patients like	Request to write policies and discuss with PCO. Check on implementation at practice visit	Audit policies, data handling, generation of letters, call and recall must be present to achieve the standards	Patient acceptance of policies often described in answer to questions on relationships with staff
Business planning	Ability to understand environment and plan for future	Requirement to involve staff in plan	Ability to self-organise to succeed, requires self-review and PDSA cycles	Indirectly in quality of service and directly with small group or by survey for specific purposes
Learning from experience/risk management	Constant improvement to a learning organisation	Significant event audit	Change in organisation required to achieve clinical standards Managing chronic illness reduces risk of premature death	Not examined
Health and safety	Use of appropriate equipment in a safe environment for staff and patients	General requirement and specific task monitoring, equipment monitoring	Not examined	Not examined
Financial integrity	Protection from fraud or non-payment of wages	Checking on who authorises what payment for staff, not partners	Not examined	Not examined

Audit	Ability to look at local process for many parameters not in the contract	Single audit required	Ability present if disease audits produced	Not examined
Medicine management				
Prescribing	Recording and appropriate use of prescribing with monitoring for side effects	Presence of record of drugs Formulary acceptance, repeat prescription availability, some batch no and expiry date recording, group directions for non-doctors. Discussion of and review of prescribing with advisor	Use of certain drugs in specific clinical areas	Not examined
Medication review	Presence of a contact to check appropriate, monitor and remove redundant prescribing. Interactions and side effect monitoring	Presence of a medicine review	Detailed examples audited	Not examined
Premises				
Premises	Multiple expansions to make fit for purpose as ascends quality ladder	Physical check on premises to baseline requirements	Larger premises have to be present to house all the staff	Are they comfortable and functional?

* In organisational domain, contractual and statutory requirements and additional services

Table 8.3 Significant areas left out of the Quality and Outcomes Framework.

Area of care	Remarks
Patients with multiple illnesses	Patients have more than one illness at a time. The requirements of treatment for one disease may conflict with another. Measuring the quality of the decision-making process to move away from a guideline is difficult
Terminal illness	Includes malignant disease but also includes LVD, neurological and other diseases
Malignant disease	There is a clinical criterion for malignant disease but much more could be achieved by using a different method. This could review care from concern about a symptom to diagnosis and support during curative and palliative treatment
Mental illness	Managing and treating some illness, supporting patients receiving care elsewhere and crisis management. Review of screening uptake and encouragement of patients to participate in standard screening programmes
Learning disability	Review of physical problems and provision of support, encouragement to participate in specific and standard screening programmes
Carers	Including in decision-making process where appropriate. Valuing their contribution to healthcare and meeting their support needs

Chapter 9

Assessment and improvement of quality

The practice visit

The Quality and Outcomes Framework contains criteria that can be measured now but this may become easier as IT systems are changed to facilitate some of the measurement. The practice will collect specified data for each criterion. For many criteria this will mean a computer search and the production of the report or transcription of the result. The guidance clarifies these issues for each individual criterion.[41] The requirement to discuss managerial issues and to look at clinical work and notes means that the visitors will include managerial and clinical representation from the PCO. The frequency of the practice visit will be determined by the speed with which it wishes to climb the framework. The expectation is of an annual visit. Once a practice has achieved most organisational standards then written (mostly computer) data can be used to decide that year's payment and the visit frequency can be reduced.

A few criteria, like the quality of notes entries, need to be checked on the day. It is intended that the supporting evidence will allow the visit to take place on one half-day for all four domains with some discussion of the next year's objectives and infrastructure requirements.

There is not enough time to check every criterion on the visit but a reserve power exists to look at all criteria if it emerges that the practice is misrepresenting its achievement. The clarity of the criteria is intended to eliminate misunderstanding and prevent this happening. This will also have the effect of reducing the number of appeals because the practice will know whether it has achieved the standard.

The effectiveness of a practice will be based on the use the practice makes of the professionals and staff within it. The learning and job plans of the practice will profoundly affect what can be achieved. The PCO will review the collective document (practice development plan) that lists which skills are available or to be developed in the future. This forms a significant element of the visit and future planning.

It is not anticipated that the visit would be the only contact with the PCO during the year. However, on a visit when the practice and the PCO are present there is an opportunity to discuss expected development in the next year. The practice is expected to improve each year until steady-state levels are reached. Even then, there may be discussion of additional and enhanced services, IT developments and premises. The core task of the visit is an assessment but, as with any other scheme, other tasks could be discussed.

Achieving a high number of points or improvement from a low level on the Quality and Outcomes Framework is difficult and worthy of managerial and peer congratulation. Improvement in quality of clinical care and organisational development reflects well on PCO managers.

The number of organisational criteria to be measured will increase as practices improve their performance. Visits will need to be tailored to the level reached. Once the contract is in operation there will have been previous assessments that looked at other practice systems. It is hoped that the statutory requirements will not provide problems for practices performing well on the contract. However, some of the statutory criteria are likely to change with time. For example, the requirement to meet Health and Safety and instrument decontamination requirements has in the past undergone rapid change, leaving many with inadequate systems.

The ability of the practice to vary workload and ask the PCO to provide some services will require discussion. For example, a practice that is in difficulties with recruitment and achieving the Quality and Outcomes Framework may choose to ask the PCO to provide some services for them. This could either mean stopping nationally enhanced services or asking the PCO to provide additional services. Conversely, a practice that has the infrastructure and personnel may wish to take on new enhanced services. The practice will need to assess its own workload but the PCO will have an overview of the local area and solutions used elsewhere.

Using formative external schemes

The summative criteria used in the frameworks do not of themselves produce improvement. The practice has access to increasing resources as quality improves. Practices can be isolated and do not necessarily know how others are achieving the same tasks. The formative quality schemes provide a mechanism that practices can use to obtain peer review of their systems. Some existing formative quality schemes overlap the new contract organisational standards. Practices could participate in these schemes as a method of climbing the quality hierarchy by being taught or helped to learn the skills necessary to succeed. Quality Team Development (QTD) from the RCGP is similar to the contract but entirely formative. It is already purchased by many PCOs to help practice development.

The Quality Practice Award (QPA), also from the RCGP, has similar criteria and standards to the Quality and Outcomes Framework and also contains formative and summative elements. A QPA pass requires the vast majority of criteria and several more have been met at a high standard. Further work will decide how achievement of this external standard will result in less monitoring and automatic acceptance for some criteria.

Other schemes, like Membership by Assessment of Performance (MAP) and Fellowship by Assessment (FBA), require similar levels of achievement for individuals. They include organisational elements and personal clinical practice in peer review. The individual nature of the assessment means that they have not been recognised as a method of meeting the levels of the organisational framework. They are likely to provide the skills necessary to implement the new contract. Similarly the practice could use another organisation or quality marker or even a commercial consultancy to do the same thing. Possession of a personal quality marker by an individual does not prove that the same organisational or clinical criteria are met in any new practice the individual moves to. However, possession of these skills is likely to be of benefit to the new practice. This enables the contract to encourage GPs to attain the skills that are required to implement the Quality and Outcomes Framework.

Dealing with poor practice

The contract is intended to help the willing to improve. It is not a policing system and will not reliably reveal poor practice outside the areas in question. There is no easy way to prove if individual clinical decisions are poor or if inappropriate care is delivered.

The contract will show up where organisational development is poor and provide information to the PCO about many activities. Practices that choose not to enter the Quality and Outcomes Framework are likely to be scrutinised by the PCO. However, the numbers who choose not to enter the framework at all are likely to be small.

There are many reasons why a practice would perform poorly on the framework. They are not all clinical. It is entirely possible that good clinical care will emerge where there is inadequate practice organisation. The contract provides a tool to find this and a developmental agenda to rectify it.

If the PCO has good reason to believe that the computer data and declared performance on the Quality and Outcomes Framework of a practice are incorrect, it has the ability to force a detailed inspection of the practice. This would require investigation of clinical records and is only available for suspected fraud. That part of the visit looking at records would need to be undertaken by a clinician.

If poor or dangerous practice is suspected, mechanisms to take action already exist. These are severe and unchanged by the contract. The aim of the development agenda is to provide the resources necessary to allow improvement before any remedial or disciplinary action is required. Practices access the resources for development by entering the Quality and Outcomes Framework and gaining additional resources as their performance improves.

Chapter 10

Enhanced services

These are a series of extra services that practices can choose to provide. The division of services into essential, additional and enhanced allows practices under pressure to reduce services and others to increase the breadth of service they provide. Some have been specified at national level and others can be negotiated locally.

The nationally specified services are of two types. Directed enhanced services are services GPs are expected to provide and have a right to provide should they wish to do so (Table 10.1). National enhanced services (Table 10.2)

Table 10.1 Directed enhanced services and assessment methods.

Directed enhanced service	Description	Comments
Access to general medical services	A payment to fund the reduction of the access time to the national target	Funds achievement of the criteria. Once achieved, payment is through the access payment in the Quality and Outcomes Framework
Childhood immunisations	A payment to fund the achievement of childhood vaccination targets	Stepped payment for achievement of 70% and 90% targets. Exception reporting is not allowed
Influenza immunisation for those in the 65 and over and other risk groups	A payment per vaccination for patients over 65 or five specified diseases or long-stay residential care	The diseases are: • Chronic respiratory disease, including asthma • Chronic heart disease • Chronic renal disease • Immunosuppression due to illness or treatment • Diabetes mellitus
Minor surgery	A range of payments for many different minor operations	Agreement required from PCO subject to satisfactory facilities, nursing support, sterilisation, consent, pathological examination, audit and patient monitoring
Quality information preparation	A payment to fund the initial summarisation of the notes of a practice	Funds achievement of the criteria. Once achieved, payment is through the summaries payment in the Quality and Outcomes Framework
Services to staff dealing with violent patients	A payment for providing essential and other general medical services to patients identified as violent	Likely to be a service provided for an area rather than in every practice. A secure location is required in which to consult patients

Table 10.2 National enhanced services and assessment methods.

National enhanced service	Description	Assessment method
Anticoagulation monitoring	Payment for helping patients to understand the reason for treatment and monitoring medication	No assessment method in addition to appraisal
Enhanced care of the homeless	Additional payment for providing essential and other services to a difficult-to-reach population in practices with a significant number of homeless patients	No assessment method in addition to appraisal
Intrapartum care	Payment for delivering intrapartum care	Annual audit of care and Diploma of Royal College of Obstetricians or experience
Intrauterine contraceptive device (IUCD) fitting	Payment for fitting and review of IUCD	Experience and up-to-date appropriate family planning letter of competence. Formative audit of care required
Minor injury service	Payment for a service that falls between essential services and severe injuries	Experience and education and audit reviewed through appraisal
More specialised services for patients with multiple sclerosis	Payment for regular review of patients and contact with specialist services	Experience and appraisal
More specialised sexual health services	Payment for testing and screening for sexually transmitted illnesses and provision of condoms and pregnancy testing. Contact tracing	Experience and education with specific formative audit and appraisal
Patients who are alcohol misusers	Payment for creation of a register and acute and supportive treatment of alcohol misusers	Formative annual review, experience and appraisal
Patients suffering from drug misuse	Payment for creation of a register and acute and supportive treatment of drug misusers	Formative annual review, experience and appraisal
Provision of near patient testing	Payment for call and recall of patients on five specific drugs for monitoring	Formative annual review, experience and appraisal Reporting and review of deaths whilst on treatment
Provision of immediate care and first response care	Payment for assistance to paramedic ambulance services in specified locations	Specialist qualification and following the local rules of the emergency service. Annual driving tuition and 5-yearly medical training
Specialised care of patients with depression	Payment to allow improved training and more time for depressed patients	Formative annual review, experience and appraisal

have a nationally set description and assessment arrangements but the PCO can decide whether it wants to contract with practices or other organisations. The difference between directed and national enhanced services is whether PCOs are required to allow GPs to offer the service.

In addition, PCOs can contract directly with practices to create locally enhanced services. The specification would be local and the assessment method and quality assurance a local decision.

References

(NB: relevant websites given at first mention)

1 NHS Confederation and BMA (2003) *New GMS Investing in General Practice*. NHS Confederation and BMA, London.
2 Royal College of General Practitioners (2001) *RCGP Information Sheet No 8: the structure of the National Health Service*. Royal College of General Practitioners, London. www.rcgp.org.uk
3 Department of Health (2001) *Shifting the Balance of Power within the NHS: securing delivery*. Department of Health, London.
4 McColl A, Roderick P and Gabbay J (1998) Performance indicators for primary care groups: an evidence based approach. *BMJ*. **317**: 1354–60. www.bmj.com
5 Capewell S, Pell J, Morrison C *et al.* (1999) Increasing the impact of cardiological treatments: how best to reduce deaths. *Eur Heart J.* **20**: 1386–92.
6 Department of Health (1999) *Saving Lives: our healthier nation*. Stationery Office, London.
7 Department of Health (2000) *The NHS Plan: a plan for investment, a plan for reform*. Stationery Office, London. www.nhs.uk/nhsplan
8 Audit Commission (2002) *A Focus on: general practice in England*. Audit Commission, London.
9 Medical Practices Committee (2002) *Final Annual Report 1948–2002*. Medical Practices Committee, London. www.open.gov.uk/dok/mpc/mpch.htm
10 Royal College of General Practitioners (2001) *RCGP Information Sheet No 1: profile of UK general practitioners*. Royal College of General Practitioners, London.
11 British Medical Association (2001) *National Survey of GP Opinion*. British Medical Association, London.
12 BMA Scotland (2001) *The Reality Behind the Rhetoric*. BMA Scotland, Edinburgh.
13 Audit Commission (2002) *Recruitment and Retention: a public service workforce for the twenty first century*. Audit Commission, London.
14 Sibbald B and Young R (2001) *The General Practitioner Workforce 2000: workload, job satisfaction, recruitment and retention*. National Primary Care Research and Development Centre, University of Manchester, Manchester. www.npcrdc.man.ac.uk

15 Sibbald B, Enzer I and Konrad B (1998) *General Practitioners' Work Satisfaction in 1998*. National Primary Care Research and Development Centre, University of Manchester, Manchester.

16 D'Souza M and Lewis R (2001) Prodigy and the delivery of guidelines. *Good Clin Pract J.* **8** (5): 18–21.

17 National Primary Care Research and Development Centre (2000) *National Evaluation of First Wave NHS Personal Medical Services Pilots*. National Primary Care Research and Development Centre, Manchester.

18 United Kingdom Parliament (1992) *The National Health Service (General Medical Services) Regulations*. HMSO, London.

19 Department of Health (1997) *The New NHS: modern, dependable*. Stationery Office, London.

20 Department of Health (1998) *A First Class Service: quality in the new NHS*. Health Service Circular HSC 1998/113. Department of Health, London.

21 Marshall M (1999) Improving quality in general practice: qualitative case study of barriers faced by health authorities. *BMJ.* **319**: 164–7.

22 National Primary Care Research and Development Centre (1998) *Practice-based Planning and Review: case studies of five GP practices*. National Primary Care Research and Development Centre, Manchester.

23 NHS Centre for Reviews and Dissemination (1999) Getting evidence into practice. *Effective Health Care.* **5**: 1–16.

24 East Kent Health Authority (1998) *Primary Care – Clinical Effectiveness (PRICCE)*. East Kent Health Authority. www.kentandmedway.nhs.uk/ professional_pages/clinical_governance/welcome_to_pricce/ek_clinical_ governance_system/pricce.asp

25 Freeman AC and Sweeney K (2001) Why general practitioners do not implement evidence: qualitative study. *BMJ.* **323**: 1100–2.

26 Wilkinson E, McColl A, Exworthy M *et al.* (2000) Reactions to the use of evidence-based performance indicators in primary care: a qualitative study. *Qual Health Care.* **9**: 166–74.

27 Ferlie E, Fitzgerald L and Wood M (2000) Getting evidence into clinical practice: an organisational behaviour perspective. *J Health Services Res Develop.* **5**: 96–102.

28 Freeborn D (2001) Satisfaction, commitment, and psychological wellbeing among HMO physicians. *Western Journal of Medicine.* **174**: 13–18. www.ewjm.com

29 Demming W (1995) *The New Economics*. Massachusetts Institute of Technology, Boston, MA.

30 Drucker PF (1999) *Management Challenges for the 21st Century*. Butterworth-Heinemann, Oxford.

31 Handy C (1978) *Gods of Management*. Arrow Business Books, London.

32 Handy C (1989) *The Age of Unreason*. Arrow Business Books, London.

33 Seddon ME, Marshal MN, Campbell SM *et al.* (2001) Systematic review of studies of quality of clinical care in general practice in the UK, Australia and New Zealand. *Qual Health Care.* **10** (3): 152–8.

34 National Primary Care Research and Development Centre (2000) *The PRICCE Project*. National Primary Care Research and Development Centre, Manchester.

35 Spooner A, Chapple A and Roland M (2001) What makes British general practitioners take part in a quality improvement scheme? *J Health Services Res Develop.* **6**: 145–50.

36 Coleman T, Wynn AT, Stevenson K *et al.* (2001) Qualitative study of pilot payment aimed at increasing general practitioners' anti smoking advice to smokers. *BMJ.* **323**: 432–5.

37 Royal College of General Practitioners (2002) *Quality Practice Award: version 7.* Royal College of General Practitioners, London.

38 National Primary Care Development Team (2001) *Advanced Access in Primary Care.* National Primary Care Development Team, Manchester.

39 Commission for Health Improvement (2003) *Clinical Governance Reviews: information about primary care trusts.* Commission for Health Improvement, London. www.chi.gov.uk/eng/cgr/pct/index.shtml

40 British Medical Association (2002) *Your Contract, Your Future.* British Medical Association, London.

41 NHS Confederation and BMA (2003) *New GMS Investing in General Practice. Supporting Documentation.* NHS Confederation and BMA, London.

42 Campbell SM, Hann M, Hacker J *et al.* (2001) Identifying predictors of high-quality care in English general practice: observational study. *BMJ.* **323**: 784–7.

Part 3

Succeeding with the contract

Chapter 11

What do successful practices do?

Practices will now control their own working environment and use that control to provide locally appropriate services to patients. Improved systematic care of disease with a patient focus will be required. Practices will have autonomy and resources to improve patient care. Now comes the hard part – GPs and their practices have to deliver on that agenda. There is every reason to believe they will be successful, as they have been in the past.

GPs currently run practices as partnerships. They will need to learn the skills of a professional managing a business as the accountants and lawyers have already done. Success will require strategic management skills as well as clinical skills. It is possible and has been done by some doctors and practices. Progressively this section will describe the characteristics of practices that have already achieved the change.

Subsequent chapters will discuss the actions that need to be taken to improve a practice. The steps are not difficult but each requires continuing attention over time. Decisions need to be taken in good time and the relationship between different parts of the practice considered as decisions are taken. This journey cannot be accomplished with a single change. Time and review are required to produce a radically different organisation. GPs cannot and should not do all the management themselves. They will need to delegate but strategic management by the GPs means developing an understanding of what is happening in the practice and creating the environment for others to flourish.

Three levels of practice

The contract is not divided into levels. Improvement requires the development of skills to perform tasks. In order to explain that journey, it is helpful to use three levels to detail the changes. These are labelled as base, improving and steady state.

This section aims to describe the characteristics of types of practices.

Characteristics of a base level practice

Any description of a base level practice must be a generalisation. The description is not intended to denigrate this type of practice as many patient services can be delivered and delivered well in this environment. It is representative of the state of development of most practices 15–20 years ago.

The characteristic feature of the practice is its focus on reactive care to patient request alone. The organisation is small and employs few people but the number of doctors can vary. Some single-handed practices are like this, many are not. The doctor is available at regular times and there is a minimum number of staff to facilitate this contact. The staff are employed by and relate to the doctor directly. Whilst there could be contracts of employment and appraisal, the main method of review and development is direct personal contact. Services depend on the presence of the doctor as there are few other staff. Consequently the practice can be closed for several hours during the day with telephone contact to the doctor or a telephonist elsewhere. Emergency medicine is provided but probably in the patient's home or at an on-call centre. The surgery is not always staffed. Where the number of doctors is small, the commitment to emergency care all day every day will encourage use of communal on-call arrangements through a co-operative or deputising service.

Paper notes are likely to be used. There may be a computer system but it may only be used for registration and not for consultations. Consequently there is no database and no computerised disease register. Records and registers could exist but each is separate and can be searched by disease but not cross-linked for searches. Patient relations can be excellent and the doctor may know and greet each one as an individual. A good knowledge of medicine allows early diagnosis and speedy referral for treatment.

The practice does not have facilities to manage the diseases found in a systematic way. If patients come back they are seen and appropriate treatment and advice given. This is not methodical and there is no possibility of finding what has been done or specifically targeting the patients who default from treatment. The doctor's time is limited and there are no support services to share the load. The workload is biased towards acute illness. Each consultation is short and the pressure of expectation encourages prescriptions for each illness. The patient is 'trained' over time to see the doctor for minor illnesses and repeatedly attends for this kind of problem. Social support for those who ask for it is provided. Preventive medicine is opportunistic; a measurement of BP or weight may take place but there is no case finding of illness in populations. The nurses see patients for dressings or nursing tasks but do not extend their role into managing chronic disease.

Box 11.1   A description of a base level practice

- Number of doctors – 4
- Number of nurses – 1 wte
- Number of receptionists – 4 wte
- Secretary
- Management – administrator (recording accounts data, arranging payments, etc.)
- Opening hours – 5 mornings and 4 afternoons per week but closed for lunch time
- IT – repeat prescription system and some but not all acute prescribing, no morbidity data (BP or significant diagnoses) or disease index recorded
- Call and recall of diseases – no database and not done
- Medicine reviews – occurring with recording of data in paper notes
- Staff review and training – no formal system, unchanging practice, no need to develop staff as tasks don't change. Minimal appraisal and no internal education meetings
- Patient relations – good informal relations, no formal system of consulting patients' views and short consultations
- Business planning – good financial control, tight control of low expenses but no plan for major investment or infrastructure
- Premises – small and not easily capable of expansion

Characteristics of an improving practice

The practice is larger and has more people and more grades of staff working from the building. It is used to change and handles many tasks. New people are often hired and there are still new tasks for them to do. Records and registers are in place and increasingly computerised. Some staff know how to use the computer audit facilities and can run audits and searches of patients requiring systematic management of illness. Nurses and other clinicians will be in post and running disease management clinics. As there are new tasks to be accomplished, individual members of staff who wish to develop themselves can take on new responsibilities and learn new skills.

Management is done by different methods now and the role of the management is increasingly important. There will be a manager who has autonomy to make decisions but the tasks may be divided among a number of people, including GPs and others outside the practice.

The manager runs many of the routine processes and the staff for the partners. The doctors can manage the practice by speaking to individuals, requesting new tasks and direct involvement in clinical tasks. The original work of creating processes was done some time before and systems have to be changed again and again for new challenges. The building is larger and it is open longer.

The larger number of staff has brought new responsibilities. Staff have been employed to look after the personnel functions of the practice. Someone will be collecting information on overtime, arranging cover for the staff with holidays and sickness. Accounting for the income of the practice, paying staff, completing pension returns and income tax payments is now a significant amount of work. Someone, usually the manager, has to conduct reviews (appraisals) with the staff to review progress and understand and solve staff difficulties.

Box 11.2   A description of an improving practice

- Number of doctors – 4
- Number of nurses – 2 wte
- Number of receptionists – 4 wte
- Secretary – 1 wte
- IT staff – 1
- Management – manager and formal structure of partners, administrator (recording accounts data, arranging payments, etc.)
- Opening hours – 5 mornings and 4 afternoons per week
- IT – repeat prescription system, all acute prescribing, morbidity data added in consulting room (BP or significant diagnoses, etc.), disease indexes recorded
- Call and recall of diseases – database used for some diseases
- Medicine reviews – occurring with recording of data on computer
- Staff review and training – formal system, development of staff for specific purposes. Appraisal but no internal education meetings
- Patient relations – good informal relations, no formal system of consulting patients' views and longer consultations
- Business planning – good financial control, tight control of moderate expenses but no plan for major investment or infrastructure
- Premises – larger but still difficulty fitting people in

As a separate change but influenced by the same development, the complexity will produce a situation where no one individual or group of individuals can know what is happening. It is necessary to appoint and trust others to deal with staff or other tasks on behalf of the doctor. Personal observation no longer gives sufficient information and new systems to report on activity are required. These in their turn take people to run them and time to assimilate and understand the output. The strategic manager moves away from personal control to managing through others. The practice needs methods to specify management tasks and distribute them to the manager and partners within the practice. There is a need to meet and explain change on a regular basis, leading to decisions which are implemented by individuals on behalf of the partnership.

The management structure is likely to mean regular meetings of the partners and manager with prepared agendas. Individual areas of the practice could be allocated to individual partners as responsibilities. The partners would learn more about that area and be the first port of call for the manager on new issues involving that area. The partner responsible would present ideas and solutions to the partnership for decisions. Once decisions were made the responsible partner would implement change in conjunction with the manager who would do most of the implementation. The partner would support the manager in that role.

Box 11.3   An example of a practice management structure

Decision-making body – partnership meeting with manager
Individual responsibilities
- Partner A
  Staff – employment, contracts, appraisal, etc.
  Health and safety
- Partner B
  Finance – understanding cash flow, profitability, liaising with
    accountant
  GP training
  Clinical areas, disease management clinics, etc.
- Partner C
  Partnership agreement
  Property
  Business plan
- Partner D
  Computer systems
  Patient participation group
  Complaints

Maintaining the steady-state practice

When the practice achieves each organisational or clinical goal it can congratulate itself on a job well done. However, the management focus and resources soon move on to other areas and the individuals looking after the area have to maintain the gains. Other systems will be designed around the job being achieved in a specific way. If it is changed there will be consequences elsewhere in the practice.

As the task nears completion in every area, systems for the ongoing business are required. This changes the requirements of the service. The task is no longer to achieve change but to retain the improvement achieved. As there is no new investment in new personnel or new tasks, this cannot be used to motivate employees. Staff have to be moved around to maintain the service within fixed budgets. The service has to be maintained whilst making changes.

Even though a steady-state level has been reached, medicine advances rapidly and new challenges, new developments and new money are likely to be available over the longer term. It is this requirement to maintain a steady state that can be identified as a separate and third level. The two extremes of management style are described separately.

Significant amounts of partner time are required to manage the practice. This is not day-to-day management, which has been delegated. Time is required for meetings, understanding what the manager is doing, designing and reviewing clinical practice and protocols. This can either be an extra job for the partners or taken out of the clinical time with patients. When clinicians, usually nurses, have a patient who doesn't fit the protocol they will need to ask somebody. This requires an additional level of knowledge across many specialties. The level of clinical expertise required of the GP increases although they are no longer routinely seeing patients, which means that they need to keep up their clinical skills. This requires additional training and knowledge, which is regularly updated to give this high level input.

Command and control: cost-cutting model

One way to do this is to assume nothing will change and that once systems are in place and running, they should remain static. One potential difficulty is that the people who set up and understand the task will leave or move elsewhere in the organisation. They then need to be replaced by someone who can fulfil the same task in the same way. There is a necessity to write down everything they formerly did and the methods used as a manual for the job. Someone new is selected. It is important to find the same skills to allow the same task to be achieved. However, the hard work has been done in developing the task. The new person is not necessarily motivated to change the job and isn't encouraged to do so. The system then needs to find markers of achievement of the task. Annual review of the individual cannot be focused around improvement because none is required so it focuses on the control mechanisms and the deficiencies uncovered.

The role of the manager is to enforce compliance and obtain more tasks for the same or less money. This is understood and dominates the relationship with the staff. The proportion of business time and resources devoted to checking gradually increases and new development and change stop. The cost of the business does fall and standards are maintained at a moderate level. If they fall too far the information systems highlight this and new systems can be created. Logically the new system is then planned centrally and the individuals hired or fitted into the framework. Mistakes are avoided because there is no latitude to make them and if they occur it is because the rules were not followed and consequently they are the employees' fault.

Alternatively the task could be specified and given to an individual or group to sort out and implement. That group would see the blocks to development and produce change, hopefully successful. Once they did, the system would take over again and codify the resulting policy and cost control would begin again.

Education and training are part of the planning process and specified centrally. As the skills required are specified, they can be allocated between individuals and the cost of training reduced by only purchasing relevant training for the current job role. Networking is important and meetings are organised to allow people to get to know each other and swap information.

This replicates a similar system described earlier as control of process which denies staff the opportunity to use their skills. Nonetheless practices who manage staff have to decide between allowing staff freedom and not knowing what is happening and overburdening staff with systematic controls. There may well be specific tasks or individuals where each approach is successful; the skill is in choosing the right job specification for the right person in an appropriate part of the system.

Box 11.4 A description of a practice in steady state – command and control

- Number of doctors – 4 partners and 2 salaried doctors
- Number of nurses – 3 wte
- Number of receptionists – 5 wte
- Secretary – 1 wte
- IT staff – 2
- Management – manager and formal structure of partners, administrator (recording accounts data, arranging payments, etc.)
- Opening hours – 5 days per week
- IT – repeat prescription system, all acute prescribing, morbidity data added in consulting room (BP or significant diagnoses, etc.), disease indexes recorded
- Call and recall of diseases – database used for all diseases
- Medicine reviews – occurring with recording of data on computer
- Staff review and training – formal system, development of staff for specific purposes. Appraisal and internal education meetings. Formal control mechanisms
- Patient relations – good informal relations with a formal system of consulting patients' views and longer consultations
- Business planning – good financial control, tight control of moderate expenses with a lot of investment, a plan for future investment and infrastructure
- Premises – larger, more than one consulting room per doctor and nurse

---

The number of staff is greater and management and educational structures are slightly better developed than in the improving practice. The difference is in function. As staff and partners are no longer developing new systems, the existing appraisal and control systems dominate the time of the manager and staff. There are now more internal systems to control and they are all dependent on decisions from the manager or partners. Much time is devoted to sorting and arbitrating on individuals' problems. Partners or the manager make decisions about all aspects of the practice and, without a decision, nothing happens.

Learning organisation

The alternative strategy is to continue to involve staff in the change process and to encourage them to continue to look at their work and systems to try to improve results further. This is easy when performance has a lot of scope to improve but more difficult at steady state. It may well be that the practice itself has to develop new ideas or theories to improve further. It then needs to use more formal methods to decide if there is improvement. Some decision making is consciously devolved to staff who are encouraged to put forward suggestions for change but the responsibility rests with the partners and practice managers. There is a difficult balancing act of encouraging contributions whilst the partners retain responsibility and ensure that the quality of the service is good.

PDSA cycles will still be required to develop the service further. The simple audits and reviews of performance used to assess rapid progress may not have sufficient statistical power to tell if a true improvement has been made. Staff and doctors will need access to the current literature to see if there are known solutions for the problem. As skills develop, this becomes research. There is also the possibility that the change introduced could result in a reduction in performance. For the doctor or manager responsible for the system, this is worrying because control is lost and mistakes can be made for which the partners are ultimately responsible.

It is difficult to run an organisation where all parts are looking at new developments. Each one is likely to impact on the rest of the routine service to be delivered to patients. Co-ordination becomes a problem and structures have to be put into place to allow interpersonal contact with those managing the business. Direct contact between others is also required, leading to interactions and the spread of new ideas.

Team meetings are required to enable staff to have their say and sort out issues between themselves. As the ability of one guiding individual to understand every process reduces, the staff need to understand and organise their own training requirements. The practice needs to understand what is required of it and allocate tasks to individuals. This applies both to managing the tasks and the skills required. The business plan of the practice will list what is to happen managerially and the education plan (practice professional development plan – PPDP) will detail the educational tasks. These are important active documents in the learning practice. It takes time away from clinical work to understand what is required of the business and to plan how it will achieve the challenges it has been set or sets itself.

The NHS notices the presence of all these skills and there are requests to help others on an area basis and from professional organisations. The partners' clinical time has already been reduced to manage the practice. Involvement in external issues leads to a further reduction in the time available. The job becomes one of understanding how to motivate others inside and outside the practice and helping them with clinical problems.

> **Box 11.5** A description of a practice which is a learning organisation
>
> - Number of doctors – 4 partners and 2 salaried doctors
> - Number of nurses – 3 wte
> - Number of receptionists – 5 wte
> - Secretary – 1 wte
> - IT staff – 2
> - Management – manager and formal structure of partners, administrator (recording accounts data, arranging payments, etc.)
> - Opening hours – 5 days per week
> - IT – repeat prescription system, all acute prescribing, morbidity data added in consulting room (BP or significant diagnoses, etc.), disease indexes recorded
> - Call and recall of diseases – database used for all diseases
> - Medicine reviews – occurring with recording of data on computer
> - Staff review and training – formal system, development of staff for specific purposes. Appraisal and internal education meetings. Formal control mechanisms. Time to discuss the purpose of the practice and plan a response. Delegation of responsibility for tasks. Regular co-ordination meetings with staff, doctors and nurses
> - Patient relations – good informal relations with a formal system of consulting patients' views and longer consultations
> - Business planning – good financial control. Expenses treated as costs of the organisation and budgets for staff education and training with a lot of investment. There is a plan for future investment and infrastructure
> - Premises – larger, more than one consulting room per doctor and nurse
> - External responsibilities – now actively involved with external organisations and senior managers and partners assessing, evaluating and training others

What does it feel like to work in these organisations?

A base level practice has not changed for some time and can continue to run without stress. The difficulty is that, increasingly, the outside structure of the NHS is putting pressure on it to change. The change to payment based on achievement of outcomes will expose this practice to a loss of income. The increase in general practice funding may mean that it continues to maintain the income but improvements in resources and quality will require substantial change. This is unsettling for a practice that is unused to change. It will be necessary to develop progressively over a number of years to reach the standards expected.

An improving practice has an enormous amount of activity to control and this may be creating stress in the practice. Although change is accepted, individuals are likely to have different ideas and compromise is required. Even without severe difficulties and partnership splits, the stress of disagreement with respected colleagues is difficult. If the partners are trying to complete a full schedule of clinical work and perform management and improvement functions in their spare time, they will be under stress and feel their workload is very high.

In the steady-state practice which attempts to control the workforce, all the decisions of the practice come back to the partners and manager. This is difficult and the day job is continually interrupted by the demands of others. If a full clinical commitment is being attempted the responsibility and workload become very high. If it is successful and the results of the practice are good, this may provide motivation and professional pride to offset against the high workload. Only if the clinical task is reduced and the management task delegated does the amount of time spent on practice issues reduce. Even in this situation the intensity of the work is high.

The commitment and effort required for a learning organisation are no different. The tasks are delegated but it is still necessary to observe what is happening in the clinical and managerial arenas. Other people have day-to-day control but responsibility rests with the partners and, when there are problems, intervention by reducing the autonomy of staff or employed doctors is difficult and stressful.

The role and responsibility of partners diverge from other doctors in the practice. As the practice devolves work to other clinicians, the role of all doctors changes from the person who does things to one who oversees and answers questions for other clinicians. In time, this often results in some degree of specialisation within the practice. The partners carry additional responsibility for the environment of the practice and supervising others. Their clinical commitment has to reduce to allow this.

The contract with the PCO is held by the practice. If the salaried staff leave or become ill, the responsibility for providing the service falls on the partners. One of the responsibilities of a partner is to keep the service going if there are problems with the supporting staff.

The responsibilities of being a partner are balanced by the increased income and status. Systematic control of chronic disease does take more people and more effort. The benefits are felt by the patients and the NHS through reduced use of secondary care.

Chapter 12

Changes required to be successful

Moving from base level to improving practice

The difference between base and improving practices is the number of tasks carried out. In order to increase the number of tasks, the practice will need to plan improvement in a service and implement it. Practices now have a series of tasks to perform in the Quality and Outcomes Framework and the contractual and statutory requirements, which have to be the priority if they are not already being accomplished. In order to make the change process manageable, it is necessary to break down the task into a series of smaller tasks.

For each task there is a need to understand what is happening now and what change is required. In order to do this, there needs to be agreement in the practice about how to improve, a method to produce improvement and somebody responsible for making change happen. In time staff need to be employed and trained. Planning involving the staff will lead on to implementation. A single criterion may require several changes or several may be grouped together as one task, for example grouping the diabetes tasks together in one clinic. Once implemented, the suggested solution will need refinement. By this natural process, practices will start to use PDSA cycles.

Preparing to implement a PDSA cycle for each practice change

- Realistic appraisal of current situation (benchmarking)
- Common aim in the practice to improve
- List of tasks to perform
- Appoint person to be responsible for managing the task
- Find someone from existing staff or appoint someone new to do the task
- Appoint new staff
- Induction training and specific task training
- Plan new service (PLAN)
- Run new service (DO)
- See if the new service works (STUDY)
- Observe improvement (ACT)

The number of tasks required can be calculated by using the tools in the tool box section of the book. For contractual and statutory requirements, clinical and organisational domains, the practice can use the tool to understand which tasks they are already achieving, what they need to do and allocate responsibility to individuals. Once this has been done, if the list is large it will be necessary to prioritise which tasks should be achieved in the next year. For each new task or criterion added, it will be helpful to consider a PDSA cycle.

Once change has occurred in one area the practice can move on to modify other areas. The cycle needs to be repeated for the remaining tasks. This becomes difficult because of fatigue and the necessity for individuals with different views to work together. The most difficult part of the change process becomes convincing colleagues. The work can be shared out and time given to colleagues to agree to new ideas. Successful practices are the ones that find ways to get on despite the stress of change.

The views of others need to be considered. Problems should be solved rather than trying to enforce particular processes. There is no correct way to run a practice but sometimes change has to be forced and people may be upset. It is better to avoid this and encourage an understanding of the reasons why change is necessary. If there are good reasons not to change, it may be better to accept that.

Dealing with the stress of rapid change in a practice

- Rapid repeated change is stressful
- Compromise is required by all sides if decisions are to be taken
- Everyone should have their say
- Isolating an individual and enforcing change has negative consequences for relationships
- Sometimes it is better to wait to allow others to see the need for change
- The feelings of colleagues should be understood
- Use the listening skills of the consultation in the practice meeting
- Practice policies have to be agreed to be implemented
- If there is a good clinical reason for something, have a clinical discussion
- Involve colleagues in decision making
- Allow autonomy to other partners
- Openness and frank discussion is a good thing; serious arguments and festering disagreements are not

---

Common themes in development

Many of the clinical criteria require the creation of an accurate database either from scratch or from an existing register. This requires cleaning the database and adding material currently only recorded on paper. The database can then be used for call and recall and the end-of-year data for contract monitoring. This is described in more detail in Chapter 13.

More staff of various grades will be required to run the practice. As the number rises, the support mechanisms increase in complexity. These are described in more detail in Chapter 14.

Costs increase as staff are employed and investment rises. This is described in Chapter 20.

Existing and new staff require training, skills and knowledge to work in a different way. This needs to be co-ordinated for the practice. Chapter 15 covers education and training.

Many chronic diseases can be managed via chronic disease management clinics. These involve a doctor and nurses seeing patients by invitation. Each chronic disease requires the measurement and recording of certain clinical parameters on a regular basis. This can be achieved by designing a protocol and regular review by the practice nurse. The doctor and nurse jointly design the protocol, agree it with other members of the practice and implement it. Some of the administrative tasks, like writing to the patient and writing blood forms so that results are available when the patient is seen, can be organised by clerical staff. The partners are responsible for their employees and have to know what is happening in the clinic and take clinical responsibility. This implies some form of active involvement in review or audit. The nurses also require clear written protocols and patient group directions from the practice to fulfil their professional requirements.

As the call and recall system is developed, the relative proportion of patient-initiated contacts reduces and the number of chronic illness reviews increases. These reviews are complex and require longer consultations to address the patient's agenda and the doctor's agenda, to give information and to manage increasingly complex treatments. Data entry into the computer is required with each consultation and the computer has to be used extensively in real time. The doctor (and staff) enter the data directly so the overall workload increases. This complexity is assimilated into the working environment. All doctors increase their knowledge of common illnesses and share expertise for less common illnesses among the group.

Box 12.1 Example of a practice adding new systems

A practice of 6000 patients currently runs a chronic disease management clinic for diabetes and wishes to set up clinics for ischaemic heart disease, cerebrovascular disease and COPD.

Initially there was no audit occurring in the practice and the practice manager administers the computer system along with all other tasks. The computer is used for repeat prescriptions and the diabetes register but it is a new system recently installed with substantial capability. The practice manager looks after the wages calculations. The premises are large with staff office space and a spare treatment room.

At a series of meetings the practice decides it needs to employ new staff.

- One full-time administrator to run the computer and audit half time and administer the wages system and enter financial data on a computer.

- 0.5 wte nurse to run the clinic.
- Practice manager to stop running the computer but retain an overview and take on appraisal of the staff and nurses and review all staff job descriptions.
- 0.5 wte receptionist to help with increased demand on reception, files, telephone and prescriptions.
- One doctor reduces their surgeries by one to oversee the clinic and help with specific problems.
- A two-session retainer doctor is employed to help with the increased demand for GP appointments.
- All doctors agree to review the increased number of blood results.

A budget and time are allocated for training.

- Training for the nurses is arranged externally over three months organised by the PCO but paid for by the practice.
- The new IT clerk attends courses on using the practice computer system, audit and search on that system, medical summaries and practice accounting.
- The practice manager attends a day release college course on staff management.
- The responsible partner consults textbooks, attends a course and reviews current best practice in the area. Information gained is shared with other doctors in the practice in summary form.
- The nurses write a clinic protocol that is discussed and agreed with the doctor. The diabetes protocol is reviewed at the same time.

A spirometer is purchased for the practice and the PCT agrees an increase in the blood-taking capacity they provide in the practice.

The IT clerk is employed first, six months before the nursing staff. The IT clerk has training and reviews all patients with an existing relevant diagnosis for the clinic. Disease registers are created by reviewing the notes of patients on specific drugs and opportunistically improving summaries during patient medicine reviews in surgeries. For patients on the disease registers searches are performed to see if blood pressures or blood results are available. Where they are not available the patient notes are searched for information which is added to the computer.

By six months the disease indexes contain about half the patients with those diagnoses. Call and recall of patients with missing data is instigated and the clinic started.

The new receptionist is employed and trained. The clinic results in more patients coming to notice and the number of prescription items increases. As the new receptionist is settling in and finishing induction training they can assist with the increased demand for prescriptions. Some treatment changes are made by the nurses but most are referred to the doctors in ordinary surgeries.

Coping with increased complexity

A team of people needs to be hired, trained in clinical roles and involved in the design of new systems to see patients for specific tasks. Some practices will already be doing this but others will have to start from scratch. The increased number of people now interact professionally and socially without using the conduit of the doctor. They need space and time for development and they need to be observed to ensure that the task is being performed. The practice then needs a layer of management to do this on behalf of the doctor.

In order to provide the facilities needed by the staff, systems need to be created to control appointment availability and use of rooms and equipment. The complex system requires high-level, well-paid managers. They are expensive to employ and their cost is more efficiently used if it is spread across a number of doctors. The individual unit where the consultation occurs does not have to increase in size but the unit has to have access to management skills. This can be provided across a group of small units within a practice or between practices.

The non-clinical staff increase. In order to reduce the time spent on non-productive tasks, receptionists are employed to manage the patients' journey through to a consultation. Computer-literate staff are required to run the computer, deal with technical problems and administer the audits and call and recall of patients where data are missing from the record. As the practice becomes more capable it acquires a role helping and organising an extended team that works from the surgery.

Box 12.2 Managing the patient's journey through the system

A practice decides that too much of the doctors' time is taken up with minor self-limiting illness. It wishes to provide the opportunity for patients to speak to a nurse for advice. The practice has been planning the change for months and staff have been employed and trained. However, the patients still expect to see the doctor.

The change can be explained to patients by putting notices in the waiting room, explaining about the new option when patients request urgent appointments and by the doctor after a consultation if it was deemed inappropriate.

More staff are necessary to co-ordinate care with other parts of the medical system. People are required to have detailed systems for all the tasks of the practice. As multiple individuals handle tasks over an expanded working week, memory and the desire to do the job well are no longer enough. The staff required to deal with an issue are not instantaneously available and do not have time to deal with issues there and then or before the member of staff leaves for the end of a shift. Therefore message books, policies and ways of working understood by all staff are required. The number of investigations and prescriptions increases and systems need to change to cope with the increased numbers and the requirement to act on some of the results. All of this requires internal policies to make sure that work is completed every time.

Box 12.3   A system to make sure all maternity patients are correctly booked for care

The practice hosts the midwife clinic for most patients requiring antenatal care. When the patient sees the GP and wishes to register for antenatal care there is a need to write a referral and to invite the patient for a routine booking appointment for antenatal care in a designated clinic.

One member of staff who is part time and also works on reception has this responsibility. The GP dictates a referral to the clinic for antenatal care and sends an internal email from the patient record to a particular member of staff. There is a permanent record of it being sent in the computer record and the next time the member of staff uses the computer in their own name, the record of a task to do is there until it is dealt with. They can deal with it when they next have appropriate time available without the fear of forgetting to act on the request.

For maternity care, sending to an individual works. For something more urgent it could be a group of staff and the particular file would be reviewed daily by whichever staff member was doing the job that day.

System changes required for expanding services

- Procedure books developed by subject
- Systems to deal with results:
  - Bloods
  - Letters
  - Read coding diagnoses
- Prescription systems to cope with large volumes
- Complicated appointment schedules:
  - Writing
  - Implementing
  - Fitting partners and staff into them

Creating a learning organisation

Creating a learning organisation is about belief. All members of the practice have to feel that their opinion matters and is useful. The person who knows most about an individual job is the person doing it. They may not be able to design it or present changes but they will understand what they do. It is important to persuade the practice that the organisation is open to change and people will be listened to. This can be achieved by clarifying the aim of the organisation. It is best if this is based on shared values. It is then possible for the practice to have a common desire to improve. Once this is in place, a plan to reach the aim can be created and the education requirements for individuals worked out.

This is easy to say but difficult to do. Opinions will on occasion conflict and unworkable solutions could be offered. The role of the top team in a business is to absorb the difficulties and allow the staff to develop. It is necessary to understand how the practice manages itself and the current attitudes and skills. The important factors for understanding the practice management structure are listed in Tool 12.1.

Tool 12.1 Understanding the management of a practice

Who makes the decisions?

Is it a single partner?
Is it the manager?
Is it collective with all partners?
Do partners have individual areas of responsibility?
If so, what can be decided individually and what requires collective decision making?
How are meetings organised – how much preparation and explanation?
Who chairs the meetings?
How are staff involved in decision making?
How is conflict handled?
How effective are individuals at achieving change?
Is there any appraisal of the managerial role of partners?
Are managerial responsibilities equal?

How much autonomy does the manager have?

Can the manager implement agreed decisions without reference to the partners?
What tasks does the manager currently do?
Can new tasks and responsibilities be taken on?
Can existing tasks be delegated?

Clinical autonomy

Can individuals tailor care for patients?
Is there agreement about most clinical situations without protocols?
Can that agreement be written down to codify but not restrict practice?
Do protocols exist?
Are they used?
Were they agreed with those expected to use them?
How are they reviewed?
Are they routinely ignored for all patients by some staff or partners?
Do nurses see patients without close review by the doctor?
Can they make decisions based on understanding of the clinical area?

How are problems and conflict in clinical practice resolved?
Can non-doctors make suggestions for changing clinical practice or
  systems?

Communication

Are there clinical meetings of the doctors?
Are there clinical meetings of nurses and other professions as individual
  groups?
Are there collective meetings of many professionals?
Do professionals of all types meet and discuss patient issues outside
  formal meetings?
If there were a problem how would it be resolved?
Are the values of individual professional groups respected?

The method of moving to a learning organisation depends on the starting
point. Many of the attributes are present in an improving practice. Therefore to
move from there, the encouragement to develop needs to be maintained and
the co-ordination systems put in place to allow that to continue as complexity
increases and tasks start to be fully achieved. If the organisation has previously
been tightly managed then there is a need to encourage individuals to
contribute.

Individuals operating in this environment become more skilled and wish to
become more qualified and move on. This creates a need for educational
courses, qualifications and time to attend them. In time benefit accrues to the
wider NHS.

Does the doctor need to be the manager?

Creating an improving practice takes skills very different from those necessary
to be a doctor. The ability to understand medicine and the different job roles in
the organisation is likely to be present for all GPs. The desire to take time to
manage an organisation of this size and complexity may not be. It is the
harnessing of that understanding and organisational ability that creates a
successful organisation, therefore delegation and professional managers are
required. The doctors can only control the system if they provide the strategic
direction. This will happen if the individual units remain small. Consequently
some strategic management has to happen elsewhere.

Some doctors may not want control of their working day or their own
organisation for some or their entire career. This is a non-partnership role. The
role of a salaried doctor is to contribute to clinical management of patients and
the clinical decision making of the practice. Organisational tasks could be
allocated as individual tasks but the responsibility for running the practice and
the effect of the decisions rest with the partners. The partners give strategic
leadership in conjunction with one or more managers who are then asked to
implement the decisions.

There is no certainty that GPs will wish to continue that role and may pass that on to professional managers. However, the success of quality schemes rests on the direct involvement of the doctors in decision making. There is benefit in keeping the organisations small enough for doctors to feel confident to provide that strategic input. Delivering the wider strategic support is the role of the PCO.

Existing research has concentrated on the involvement of GPs in running the practice. As the practice becomes a unit that is not so dependent on doctors, the attitude of other staff grades to taking responsibility for the quality of the work at a strategic level will become important. There is no reason to think that nurses or managers will behave differently. Benefit will accrue when they are directly involved in decision making, either as partners in the practice or at other levels in the system above or below the practice.

Chapter 13

Using information technology

Information technology for the contract is a tool to help achieve quality and quality criteria. The current practice systems are well known and it is not necessary to describe them. New systems will be created but the technology will change rapidly. This discussion therefore mainly deals with how a practice can prepare itself and achieve quality. It is about the people who operate the systems and what they have to be able to do to achieve that.

Who is responsible for information technology?

PCO responsibilities

The provision of information technology is to be a PCO responsibility. The requirement for GPs to contribute to the cost of practice systems has been removed. Systems can be chosen from a number of accredited suppliers but PCOs will expect to influence the systems and how they are used. This has been done to allow integration with secondary care so that data from secondary care can be displayed on GP computer systems. This can only be done if the computer systems are integrated with a common database. Data could be entered by out-of-hours teams, secondary care, specific disease managements for individual diseases, pharmacies or intermediate care teams.

There will be a need for some GPs to change systems and many will need to use more of the capacity and features of the existing systems. The existing GP computer systems from the large suppliers can achieve all that is required for the contract with the addition of a few Read codes. The systems could be improved to allow searches for some functions that currently require manual review.

A nationally funded IT programme will provide some training for staff to use computers. The PCO will provide computer staff above the level of the practice to assist with more technical difficulties in running computer systems.

Practice responsibilities

The cost of the staff to operate the systems is a practice responsibility and is paid for out of the practice resources. It is in the nature of IT training that a lot of it is practical and will need to occur whilst doing the job in practices. Practices will have to add to the national training from their own education budgets to help staff and partners reach the required level of capability. The ability to use the practice computer system in house will profoundly affect performance on the clinical indicators. Computer staff and their skills are important to practices.

Use of a computer is not specified in contract documentation but it would be extremely difficult to achieve high levels in the clinical domain without extensive use of a computerised database in the practice. Whilst there is no necessity for practices to enter data in specific ways, it is a great deal easier to enter data accurately and in the right place using a template and the same Read code for the same illness. It is likely that computer systems will produce prompts and practices will produce protocols for how they would like data to be entered. Similarly it will be a practice decision how to clean the database and which staff members are most appropriate to do that.

The contractual and statutory requirements specify that the practice has to maintain good computer use in accordance with current legislation. This

Table 13.1   How indicators assess information technology systems and ability.

Organisational area	Development need	Organisational standards*	Clinical standards	Patient questionnaire
Disease registers	Presence of a record for case finding, audit education, changing treatment as medicine develops	Cross-collation of clinical diagnoses to repeat prescribing and review of summaries Legible records	Detailed scrutiny of a small number of registers	Not examined
Secondary prevention	Case finding, updating data, data accuracy, change in clinical practice for individual patients	Presence of registers 80% smear criteria Legible records	Achievement of outcome measures in several diseases	Not examined
Confidentiality	Holding data confidentially and informing patients about use	Caldecott guardian and the display of a notice	Not examined	Not examined
IT	Accurate disease registers and searchable database of specific parameters	Not included as this can be done without computer for individual illnesses	Databases must be present to produce data at higher contract levels	Not examined
Audit	Ability to look at local process for many parameters not in the contract	Single audit required	Ability present if disease audits produced	Not examined

* In organisational domain, contractual and statutory requirements and additional services.

requires the practice to have someone responsible for confidentiality and confidentiality has to be explained to patients. The practice must be registered for data protection and make electronic data available to the next practice for patients moving practice.

These requirements can be achieved on existing systems and they will be improved and others developed. Practice staff also require the ability to perform the following tasks and the database needs to be accurate. In order to do this, practice staff will need to improve the database and enter data for the future.

Practice IT tasks

- Cleaning the database
- Entering data recorded in notes but not on computer
- Training of professionals in data entry
- Adding the data in real time in consultations for the future
- Entering data for many illnesses at one consultation
- Training of staff in audit
- In-year audits to establish performance
- Call and recall of patients with missing data or partially controlled diseases
- Preparing data for submission at year end

Cleaning and improving existing data

In many practices data have been collected in written records and not entered on computers. If the practice has been controlling blood pressures and treating hypertension well but not recording it, the task is to improve the recording of data, not to change treatment. Experience elsewhere has shown that improving recording of missing data by searching notes can result in rapid improvements in the computer records. This is a task that can be done by the computer staff and does not require expensive clinicians.

In order to target this work it is necessary to compile a disease index on the computer and then search that group to see if the parameter, say blood pressure, has been recorded in the past year. This can then be added, if present on the paper record. If notes are being obtained for this work it is more economical to look for several parameters and update the record for diabetes, CHD and other diseases at one time. Computer records for readings measured on bloods are automatically recorded if the results are gathered over an electronic link. In time it is anticipated that other clinical parameters, like blood pressure taken in secondary care, would be added to the record directly.

> **Box 13.1** Improving the computer database by using information in the notes
>
> A practice had recently started to use a computer for data entry in consultations. Patients had previously been seen and data entered in the notes. Some doctors and nurses were more comfortable using the computer than others. The practice computer system showed that 30% of hypertensive patients had a recorded blood pressure in the last year.
>
> A member of staff reviewed the notes of the other 70% of patients full time for four weeks. Half of these patients had been seen in the last year and blood pressures were recorded for 80% of these. In four weeks' work, the practice improved the computer recording of blood pressure in hypertensive patients from 30% to 58%.

Existing disease indexes are not always accurate. Sometimes inaccurate diagnoses have been recorded in the past. If patients do not have a diagnosis it is not appropriate to treat them and record parameters. Each entry needs to be checked either from the records or in a consultation. Patients will know if they have an illness in most circumstances. This cleaning of disease indexes should be done early in the process of improvement as it avoids work later if the diagnosis is inaccurate.

Some patients with illnesses may not have a diagnosis recorded. It may be impossible to rectify this easily other than by summarising the notes. However, there has to be a reason why patients are on repeat medication. This provides a ready way of identifying patients on medication for many illnesses, for example CHD or depression.

Improving new data entry

The practice needs computers in each consulting room and they need to be used by all clinical members of staff. The skills for this are basic computer use and data entry. Many practices do this already. If a practice or individual partner finds this difficult, it will be necessary to help them improve computer skills. A questionnaire for staff to use to understand individuals' current abilities is provided in the tool box. If this shows an individual learning need, it can be added to a personal learning plan. Improving the quality of data entry will require clinicians to be able to enter data in every relevant consultation for each parameter.

It is often easier to enter the data into a template on the computer than try to remember what to add. This also encourages use of common Read codes in standard situations. The template should record the important data and not record other data of less importance that is not required for every patient. It is also helpful if the template displays whether information is available but unlikely to be recorded in the consultations; for example, the last cholesterol reading was less than 5 and four months ago. Those designing templates need to be aware of the difficulties with enforcing process by this route and allowing the option to enter data rather than forcing data entry.

If past morbidity data are entered during consultations this takes considerable time but rapidly improves disease indexes.

Box 13.2   A method of improving the quality of summaries

A practice wishes to make sure their patient summaries are accurate. A lot of work has been done already and the computer summaries are present for most patients.

A paper copy of the summary is printed and added to the patient notes. If there is time in the consultation and it is appropriate, the doctor or nurse shares the written summary with the patient. The patient is encouraged to comment on the accuracy of the summary.

Illnesses can be added or removed from the record as a result of the process.

Auditing the current situation

Once the database has been cleaned and the disease indexes reflect the number of patients with particular illnesses, the practice can start to improve clinical care. For some practices this will reveal good levels of chronic disease management and only fine-tuning will be required. Effort can focus elsewhere. For others it will reveal relatively low levels of control and action will be required.

The computer record can be used to find out which patients need to be recalled and to arrange the review (usually annual) required by many criteria. These reviews can be run in conjunction with the repeat prescription system. As medicine reviews are completed the relevant information can be collected and added to the computer. There may also be a requirement to run specific letters following specific searches and to request patients to attend the surgery or supply information. The IT requirement to do this is sufficient trained staff, an accurate database and enough terminals for someone to be able to search the database. This search can be run either in the clinical system or in a separate software system. The database cannot be improved if the names of the patients missing from the registers are not known to the practice. The skills to do this must be in the practice.

General practice provides the opportunity to integrate the care of more than one illness and many illnesses require the recording of the same parameters. There is the possibility to co-ordinate care of several illnesses at the same time and reduce the number of patient contacts and appointments.

Tool 13.1   Practice IT staff competences

Number of staff

Are these functions available in the practice?
Are they available in sufficient amounts for the new environment?

Cleaning the registers

Checking if patients have the diseases listed on the disease register
Finding patients on specific medications and illness not on registers
Summarising new notes and entering accurate disease information on the
   computer
Consistently Read coding diseases in the same place
Entering data recorded in notes but not on computer

Templates

Generating own templates or using templates created elsewhere

Using the computer search program

Identifying patients with an illness
Running a call system to invite patients for review every year or six
   months
Checking if each criterion has been measured for each disease (e.g. BP in
   angina)
Finding the name and address of patients with unmeasured criteria
Writing invitations using the list generated by the computer
Checking outcome levels for groups of patients on each disease index
Re-auditing data at future dates to check if measurement or outcomes
   improving
Run the end-of-year report for the Quality and Outcomes Framework

Confidence in the general running of the computer

Backing up data
Sorting problems
Collecting data from outside, e.g. lab reports

Computer security and confidentiality

Is there a secure area to receive faxes and data?
Is there a Caldecott guardian and are minimum standards met?

Use of non-practice computer programs

Word processing
Using the clinical resources in the practice computer

Accessing libraries and journals on the Internet
Email
Other

Training

What training have the staff had on the existing computer system?
What gaps are identified?
What training is required to meet them?

Producing the annual report

The clinical domain requires the collection and presentation of data about individual patients in a tabulated form. This will mean running a defined search pattern on the computer system. The data will be required on a certain date. The computer will be able to tell what the situation was on a particular date. The visit may not be for some time afterwards. It will not be possible to change the computer data later and affect the report.

The practice has to be able to run this report and requires the skills to do so. This should be easier than organising and running the in-year searches to improve the quality of the database and thus clinical care.

Some of the organisational standards ask for information about the computer system, confidentiality and transferring data. This is reviewed in a different way.

Using other IT programs and resources

Running the practice requires the ability to present data and communicate with others. Some search programs run better if the data are exported into other software and searches run there. Most clinicians will need to access data in electronic form from the Internet or other sources.

It is not possible to decide for individuals how much knowledge they are going to require but understanding of the office software systems available is likely to be of benefit. There is an agreement with Microsoft to license its software for use in the NHS. There is no licensing cost to the individual clinician or practice for use of these products but there is a small cost to obtain the CD-ROM or Internet connection to download the software.

Other computer applications a practice might use

Software

- Word processing
- Spreadsheet to analyse data and display results
- Email
- Presentations to other partners and staff
- Practice finances
- Internet access
- Access to medical data held electronically, e.g. CD-ROM
- Calendar to display rotas and aid planning

Hardware

- High-volume printer for large documents
- Data projector for meetings
- Digital camera for medical photographs

Chapter 14

Managing the staff

Staff should have good working conditions. There are many organisational indicators to encourage good employment practice. The practice has obligations to the staff it employs as well as to the NHS. These obligations overlap and the criteria seek to replicate good employment practice. However, this is one area where practices will have to understand developments in good employment practice and statutory change as well as NHS changes.

What is expected from the practice?

There are obligations on the practice in the contractual and statutory requirements and other provisions in the Quality and Outcomes Framework.

Practice obligations to staff

- Annual appraisals
- Written terms and conditions
- Compliance with all statutory minimum terms and conditions of employment
- Compliance with all statutory minimum employment rights and discrimination legislation
- Compliance with all statutory minimum health and safety legislation
- A manual of staff employment practices (equal opportunities, bullying and sickness absence)
- Person-specific job plans for advertised jobs
- Practice policies to prevent fraud to ensure staff income and pensions are paid

---

In addition, clinical staff will be expected to jointly develop plans and policies to demonstrate competence and to improve their skills. This is achieved by the route of annual appraisals and personal learning plans. All clinical staff will have to produce documentary evidence of their qualifications and indemnity insurance.

In order to be successful a practice will have to do much more than this. It will have to delegate work to staff members and motivate them to deliver the high-quality service that patients like. Staff have to feel wanted and respected in their new roles to do this. They will also need personal and educational support. This enhancement of their role and involvement in the running of the practice and its systems are difficult to achieve but crucial to success with the clinical criteria. If the achievement of the clinical criteria is almost completely delegated to nursing staff the practice will need the staff to perform all the tasks at all times.

Table 14.1 How indicators assess good employment practice.

Organisational area	Development need	Organisational standards*	Clinical standards	Patient questionnaire
Administrative staff		Contracts, appraisal, standard employment practices, specific job specifications		High-quality patient contact Skills to run the practice in a responsive way
Practice management staff	Employment of appropriate grades, appropriate training Personal development Respect for colleagues' skills Functional teams Appraisal	Management change agenda to reach organisational framework requirements	Achievement of criteria promotes respect for colleagues and development of complementary roles based on individual talents within a team	
Nurses		Contracts, appraisal, standard employment practices, specific training on smears, checking of qualifications, staff job specifications		Clinical and communication skills
Doctors		Publication of model contracts of employment for salaried doctors		

* In organisational domain, contractual and statutory requirements and additional services.

As a practice plans how to improve its performance it will need to decide the tasks it wishes staff to perform. This will lead it to define individuals' job roles and responsibilities.

New opportunities for staff come from delegation

In return the practice can expect staff to take on new roles and responsibilities. Administrative roles can be internally defined and delegated without reference to external agencies. However, the practice is responsible for the actions of staff and needs to understand the limits of delegation.

The situation for delegation of clinical responsibility is different. The individual clinician has personal professional responsibility for their actions. Each professional body has advice available on what can be delegated. If patient group directions are required for the administration of medicines then staff as well as partners should make sure they are present.

Managerial delegation is also possible. Postgraduate education, development of internal guidelines or systems could be delegated to employed staff. If the relative proportion of the work performed by partners reduces then it will be necessary for others to develop the clinical rules of the system. Guidelines are available from many sources and could be adapted locally. If this is a delegated task, work time will need to be provided to perform it.

Once systems and guidelines have been developed they have to be introduced into practice routine. As described earlier, this is difficult. Involving more people in the guideline-writing process will help but ultimately other professionals have to want the guideline. Whether a guideline written by a staff member is successfully implemented will depend on the power or influence that person has in the organisation.

Box 14.1 How implementing a change is influenced by other clinicians' views

A new partner is given the task of writing a policy for the management of hypertension. The partner attends a number of courses and reviews the evidence and comes to the conclusion that blood pressure (of hypertensive patients) can and should be controlled to below 140/85. In conjunction with the nurses who are to run the hypertension clinic, a policy is written and introduced after brief discussion at a practice meeting.

The other five partners and the salaried doctor did not read the protocol and feel that using multiple agents to control blood pressure is inherently wrong because it causes more harm than good. They have also seen the occasional hypotensive patients where medication had to be stopped.

Six months later, most patients have been reviewed but only 35% of patients have blood pressures in the recommended range.

Learning points

- It is just as easy to ignore practice protocols as externally imposed ones (*see* Chapter 4 and Figure 4.1)
- Clinical discussion did not take place
- Individuals in a practice have power and status and can influence the implementation of new initiatives

The new partner went back to the practice and produced the figures. The subject of the next clinical meeting of the practice was changed to hypertension. There was an open discussion of the clinical reasons for controlling blood pressure to that level. The nurses presented information on how the clinic was to run and how it could help the practice to achieve better disease control without massive increases in workload.

> The clinical worries about overtreatment were aired and some potential problems uncovered. Examples of where this had been done and the lack of clinical problems were discussed. The clinic structure and practice policy were amended slightly.
>
> The partners expressed a desire to see the next audit, which showed improvement. All partners had improved their understanding of an important and common disease and improved their care of it from a position of increased knowledge.

Disagreement in a practice at partnership level over a clinical or administrative change could mean that the task of guideline development is then allocated to a relatively junior member of staff. This person is then required to implement change either in a clinic setting or by persuading others. Not surprisingly, this doesn't produce change and causes problems for the person charged with implementing it. If this occurs it is better to acknowledge that change is not happening and for the partnership to reach agreement or to wait until the need for change becomes apparent to all staff members.

It is good practice for staff to understand their own job role and to try to improve working methods. The practice should be ready to consider any change proposed. If the staff can make the case for change it will be easier for the partnership to accept it. Therefore the ability to audit and make a case for a development is a beneficial skill for both the individual and the practice.

It is expected that the day-to-day management of the practice will be delegated to a manager or managers. This is a substantial task and responsibility that requires ability and skill. Managers should expect support from the partners and a clear description of what has been delegated. The degree of independent decision making open to the manager needs to be known for day-to-day work and strategic decisions. There is no necessity to have a manager in every individual surgery and groups of small surgeries may well develop with shared managers. In this situation the manager becomes very important to the practice and the position in relationship to the partnership changes. In time, less active GP partners with autonomous managers will have to bring them into the partnership.

What should be delegated and to whom?

The practice should consider how it would like to use its doctor time, nurse time, pharmacist time or care manager or indeed any other new professional grade to accomplish the clinical and administrative task. At present there are assumptions about what individual clinicians and staff will do. The practice now has the freedom and ability to provide those tasks in a different way.

The list of tasks to be accomplished in the practice will suggest the job description of the staff member employed for the post. Several job roles and tasks can be included in the job description of a new member of staff. The cost can then be calculated and compared with the increased income available for completion of the task. If the new job role is viable then a contract of employment and job description can be written and a new staff member employed. Once the post is up and running the job can be reviewed for effectiveness and efficiency.

The existing staff may wish to change job roles and may have valuable experience. When changes are considered it is appropriate to consider the existing structure and whether existing staff could fulfil some of the new job roles. A simple list of the staff in post and their current job roles and a questionnaire of their interests, skills and previous training will help this.

Find out from the staff what they do now and what they could do

- Current duties
- Previous training
- Existing skills
- Skills developed before and not currently being used

Many of the organisational criteria require the writing of a practice policy. The staff know their own jobs and are in a good position to write these down. With encouragement and support this can be accomplished which will give an overview to the partners and manager of what happens in the practice. Good ideas often emerge from such an exercise and some policies that require improvement may come to light. The document produced is also useful for new staff members as part of the induction process.

Tool 14.1 Policies required from the practice

Contractual and statutory regulations

In practice leaflet (CS 1)
Description of appointment system
Description of repeat prescription system
Complaints procedure (CS 2)
Consent to treatment of children (CS 6)
System to allow patients access to records (CS 11)
System to ensure data are transferred if patients leave practice (CS 13)
Procedure for the electronic transmission of data (CS 15)
Systems of clinical governance (CS 20)

Organisational domain

System for transferring and acting on out-of-hours (OOH) information
  (Records 3)
System for messages and visit requests (Records 4)
System for hospital reports and investigations (Records 5)
System for informing team members if a patient has died (Records 6)
System to alert OOH if patient is dying at home (Records 13)
Policy on what is included in a summary (Records 15 and 18)

System to contact OOH by a fixed number of telephone calls (Patient communications 1 & 8)

Written policy on telephone availability (Patient communications 3)

Written policy on removing patients (Patient communications 4)

Staff appraisal system (Education and training 8)

Management 1 Description of how local procedures accessed (Practice management 1)

Clearly defined arrangements for backing up computer data (Practice management 2)

Systems for inspection and calibration of equipment (Practice management 7)

Policy for prevention of fraud (Practice management 8)

Protocol for the identification of carers (Practice management 9)

Procedure manual including staff employment policies (Practice management 10)

Procedure to identify patients defaulting from regular neuroleptic medication (Medicines management 7)

Additional services

System to follow up abnormal/inadequate smears (Additional – CS 2)

Policy to identify and follow up smear defaulters (Additional – CS 3)

System to inform all women of smear results (Additional – CS)

Policy for auditing cervical smear service (Additional – CS 6)

Policy for responding to requests for emergency contraception (Additional – CON 1)

Policy for providing preconceptual advice (Additional – CON 2)

Note the detailed requirements are given in new GMS contract supporting documentation. The names of the organisational areas differ between documents. The names in the main contract document have been used.

Limits on delegation and staff structure

The employment of staff has to be balanced by more income or a falling workload. Practices have to consider what benefit they will achieve by employing new staff. The income is fixed by the global sum, quality payments and enhanced services and staff have to be employed from that sum.

There are limits on the number of clinical staff to employ in any area. The number of available trained nurses is limited. The rest of the NHS is competing for nurses and there is no certainty they will always be available. The same is true of GPs, both partners and salaried doctors. Reception staff are available but new staff will require training, particularly if additional responsibilities or IT skills are required.

The professional codes of practice limit what can be delegated and support is required for extending the role. The amount of support increases the cost and if it is going to be substantial, the delegation may not be economic.

Once staff are employed they need to be retained. In some areas the increase in practice staff will be substantial. This rapidly expanding job market will lead to opportunities for doctors, nurses, managers and administrative staff to move. Treating them well and maintaining an interesting job for all grades is therefore important. Delegating all the simple work from a job or limiting personal clinical contact may improve job satisfaction for some or remove the reason for doing the job in the first place.

Tool 14.2   Staff functions required in the practice

Administration

Access and appointments
Enquiries at front desk
Telephone answering
System for making and storing appointments
Booking patients in
Making prescriptions and repeat prescriptions available
Comfort of patients whilst waiting
Entertainment of patients whilst waiting (books, magazines, play area for
  children)

Consultations

Availability of rooms by rota
Patient call to the rooms
System to book further appointments, tests, minor procedures, etc.
Making notes or computer records available for the consultation

Back office functions

Clinical and administrative audit
Call and recall of patients
Managing the referral process with letters and faxes to eliminate errors
Summarising notes (existing and new to practice)

Administration

Staff contracts
Appraisal
Payroll for staff
Financial understanding (accounts, cash flow, financial predictions)

Managing

Staff
IT
Premises
Facilitating meetings and contacts between staff
Health and safety
Running the partnership (shares, voting rights, ownership of assets)
Leadership and support within the business
Control systems (when to use, when not to use)
Understanding and improving the quality of outputs from staff
Education

Supporting the increased number of staff

Employing more clinical staff has implications for the number of support staff necessary. Having more appointments and consultations will increase the number of patients attending reception and booking appointments. This is likely to require more support staff. The number of computer terminals running appointments may need to be increased and if paper records are used, more will have to be available for surgeries and filed afterwards. With increasing repeat medication comes an increase in the complexity of the repeat prescription system. More phone calls are required to change appointments and check results. The premises often become a constraint on increasing the number of patients seen.

As a practice moves from having few staff to the large number required for all these tasks then managing and paying them accurately and on time becomes a significant task in itself. Some new specialist roles become necessary for which training may be required.

As the number of staff increases it is necessary to document how well individuals are doing and how the practice can help them improve or develop new skills. The job descriptions and appraisals of staff are the tools required to run this larger organisation. They will reveal the gaps in knowledge and the training needs of individuals which will feed into their personal development plans. Expertise in reviewing and appraising staff is required.

When the practice is planning for new staff and new job roles it will have a list of the training requirements for the whole practice. This is the practice professional development plan. Deciding on that training, organising it and paying for it are practice responsibilities. The funding for this is contained in the global sum.

The practice also has to ensure that the service delivered is of a high-quality. All individuals employed have to be functioning well. This is achieved by helping staff to improve and the practice requires systems to check the quality of the work produced by clinical and administrative staff. The systems used within the practice also need to be subject to review. Systems are required to check and update quality for each of the areas in Tool 14.3.

Tool 14.3 Practice systems to encourage quality of working

Clinical

Method for writing internal guidance
Audit and control systems to reveal what actually happens
New entrants' teaching to fill the gaps found and prepare for the future
The quality of the planning and decision-making processes
Prescribing
Referrals

Administrative

Method for writing internal procedures
Audit and control systems to reveal what actually happens
New entrants' teaching (induction training)
The quality of the planning and decision-making processes

Coping with the Quality and Outcomes Framework as a non-partner

This book has focused on the role and responsibility of those who run the practice and the PCO to organise change. Most of the people working in or for a practice are not partners. As practice nurses, salaried doctors and more skilled managers are brought into the system there will be a need to understand the differences between the roles. Clinical and managerial functions will be delegated. This should be a positive experience and allow non-partners to have an influence on the business and use their knowledge to produce solutions.

Staff of all levels will need to be aware of the limits of delegation and the pitfalls of taking on tasks they cannot achieve. The structures to govern the relationship between staff and the business, job descriptions, learning plans and appraisals are their opportunity to discuss how much delegation is appropriate and their training and development needs.

Chapter 15

Education and training

This is a key area of development. If the staff and partners aren't knowledgeable and skilled at their job the most wonderful system won't work well. If they are knowledgeable and skilled they will find a way of delivering a better service by adding value even in difficult circumstances. The challenge for the practice is to enable staff members to achieve all the contract criteria and high standards for the rest of the work of the practice. A method to do this is required.

What is expected from the practice?

As the practice is free to organise itself internally to achieve the quality specification, it is not appropriate to specify here the grades and training staff must have. Once the staff member is in post, it is appropriate to work backwards to the skills they require and then the training requirement they need.

The resources for training are included in the payments made to practices. For particularly expensive courses and the development of individuals, this is a PCO responsibility. For all the rest it is a practice responsibility. The contract is structured to provide safeguards for the staff and the system by specifying standards of behaviour from practices and outcomes that should be achieved. Personal learning plans and appraisals are required for all and the practice professional development plan will be a public document and shared with staff and PCO.

Table 15.1 How indicators assess education and training.

Organisational area	Development need	Organisational standards*	Clinical standards	Patient questionnaire
Administrative staff	Knowledge, skills and attitudes to perform the job Personal development	Appraisal Three-yearly updating of basic life support skills Induction training	Achievement of criteria requires knowledge and skills	High-quality patient contact Skills to run the practice in a responsive way
Practice management staff		Management change agenda to reach organisational framework. Induction training. Review of patient complaints. Significant event review. Clinical governance system and clinical governance lead	Planning the learning needs to enable the organisation Reorganisation of training plans to achieve criteria and standards Review and change of methods when steady state reached	The overall feel of the practice through training of others
Education of nurses	Knowledge, skills and attitudes to perform the job Personal development planning Updating in the major disease areas Annual appraisal	Appraisal, personal learning plans, specific training on smears, checking of qualifications, treatment of anaphylaxis 18-monthly updating of basic life support skills Induction training	Specific learning needs for individual clinical tasks and clinics Review of the evidence base	
Education of doctors		Appraisal Induction training Personal learning plan implied in preparation for appraisal	Specific learning needs for individual clinical tasks. Doctors will often challenge clinical criteria, which leads to a review of evidence. Will require development of skills to look at the evidence base	Indirectly through ability to communicate and inform about illness

* In organisational domain, contractual and statutory requirements and additional services.

Deciding how much training is required

The old arrangements and payments (Postgraduate Education Allowance) no longer exist under the new contract. The practice collectively is responsible for the development of skills for the practice. This was already the case for the staff, including salaried doctors. This is a significant responsibility and checks and balances have been built in to review performance.

Practices will have to meet the specific education requirements to achieve the criteria. These can be worked out and sources found for each of the clinical criteria. For each there is a need to understand the reason for the criterion, how to make changes and achieve it and how to explain why to the patient. A tool listing the areas requiring attention is in the tool box (Tool 26.2). Once patients are on medications the doctor, or whoever is reviewing the patient, will need to understand the interactions and monitoring requirements of all the drugs used.

Clinical indicators

- Which diseases require improved clinical skills?
- Understanding and checking the evidence base
- Improved understanding of illnesses and expectations of treatment
- Knowledge of the diagnostic methods and treatments
- Ability to explain to patients

Medicine reviews

- Education about interactions
- Education about side effects
- Education about monitoring

The knowledge and skills required to achieve the organisational criteria are not required of every doctor in the practice. These can be allocated to individuals or groups to investigate the tasks on behalf of the practice. The requirement here is to decide if each criterion has been achieved. If not, the task is allocated to an individual or group who plan how it can be achieved by changes to practice structure and function. The education required to do this follows. This applies to the organisational changes required for the 10 clinical areas as well as the organisational domain, patient experience, additional services and contractual and statutory requirements. Tools for each area can be found in the tools section.

Organisational indicators

- Benchmarking of current activity for each indicator
- Listing skills, facilities and personnel available
- Finding the gaps
- List of educational needs for the practice
- Implementation of change – persuading staff and partners to change
- Involving staff in future development, PDSA cycles, changing structures
- When achieved, maintenance of the steady state

The list of changes to practice structure and function become the business plan and the training requirements become the practice professional development plan.

In addition, there is a broader agenda of changing the organisation and improving its function. Achieving the criteria will require the development of skills both clinical and managerial. For instance, the IT skills to run the practice and communicate using word processing and email will not be found as requirements of the Quality and Outcomes Framework but they are still important to the practice. Education will be required to continue treating other illnesses not in the framework.

Each criterion of the organisational standard requires a piece of work or the attainment of an educational task, as shown in Box 15.1.

Box 15.1 Using an indicator to reveal an educational requirement

Example: creating and maintaining contracts of employment for staff

In order to have contracts of employment for all staff, someone in the practice has to understand the details of writing contracts, the broad nature of each job role in the practice and the terms and conditions available to each employee.

They also need to have a legal background in employment law. If this is not already the case someone (probably the practice manager) would need to obtain those skills or a new person with the skills employed. The practice would discuss and agree a method of obtaining the training and the time to undertake it. The cost of the training would be a practice responsibility.

For more complex situations involving employment law the practice could take advice from external specialists in the field. This is currently available through the BMA and the PCOs, both of which have expertise.

The patient experience could produce different educational agendas. This will review the ability of all staff to communicate with patients. In order to achieve maximum points score in the whole contract the practice will have to understand how patients would like to use it. It will benefit most if the views of the whole practice population are tested. This will take skills not currently found in many practices. The questionnaires are likely to review the way the appointment and telephone systems affect patients which may have implications for systems and staff training in communication. For clinical staff the focus is likely to be aspects of the consultation technique.

Creating the practice professional development plan

This list of tasks to be accomplished for clinical, organisational and patient experience could be used as the basis for the practice education plan. They are detailed in the tool box section of the book (Tools 27.1–27.4). This is likely to be a long list of tasks, some of which everyone needs to know about and others that are allocated to individuals. This list can be transcribed or, using the computer software, cut and pasted into individual tables for each person within the practice.

Each individual then has a series of requirements. It is possible, even likely, that the list will be extensive and uneven. The practice will then have to decide which tasks have to be completed first. A timescale is then allocated. If the task requires a lot of investigation and writing up, more time will be required. For employees this time will have to be paid for. It is not a requirement for partners but taking on large amounts of additional work is likely to lead to problems and overwork. Practice time is probably required for partners too. If there is to be time out of practice it will have to be paid for. This is a cost of development. Practices that have already made the changes will not have to do this whilst those with further to travel will have to invest before they can reap the financial rewards.

The personal development plan forms the basis of appraisal. This provides the clinician with an opportunity to discuss the task they have taken on with a colleague.

Creating an education plan

- List of tasks to be accomplished (using Tools 27.1–27.4 or other method)
  - Create practice professional development plan
- Allocate to individuals
- Allocate a timescale
  - Create personal development plans
- Review progress at appraisal

The contract and particularly the clinical criteria do not cover the whole of medicine. In the first few years of the contract these clinical areas may be priorities. In time learning and experience of others will be required. The rest of clinical medicine is important and requires clinical skills too. In time the specific organisational skills can be applied by practices to new diseases.

Table 15.2 An example of the development process for the practice professional development plan.*

Organisational standard	Is it happening already?	Who should do this task?	Responsible person?	Structural change required?	Skills required?	Training/course required?
D. Practice management						
Access to local child protection policy	No policy in the library	Practice manager to request policy	Partner B	No	All clinicians to read manual and understand responsibilities	Read the manual and discussion of effect on practice or existing practice
Process to back up computer data and control the addition of programs	Back up yes Control of additional programs no	IT manager	Partner D	Writing and agreeing a policy with partner D and later the partnership	No	IT manager to discuss with IT provider which software is a potential problem
Recording of hepatitis B status and immunisation of clinicians	No	Practice manager	Partner A	Creating a database, requesting information from staff	Understanding confidentiality issues	Private study by partner and contacting medical defence organisation
Compliance with national guidelines for instrument sterilisation	Yes but steam steriliser old	Practice manager to find out if the steriliser is still adequate and plan replacement for function	Partner A	Replacing the steriliser or purchasing a sterilising service	Nil. May require some training for nurses if a new steriliser is purchased that works differently	Nil
Appointment times to patients meet minimum requirements	Yes	Nil	Partner D	No. Receptionist responsible for creating surgery rota to write down how this is done	Nil	Nil
Person specifications and job descriptions are produced for all advertised vacancies	No	Practice manager	Partner A	System to decide what is required and write person specification involving meeting between manager and partner before job advertised	Practice manager to understand legal responsibilities and pitfalls	Practice manager and partner A to attend course on employment law and purchase textbook

The practice has systems in place to ensure regular and appropriate inspection, calibration, maintenance and replacement of equipment	For some, not all	Practice manager	Partner A	Check on current service contracts and report back to practice. Organise for electrician to check electrical safety of each appliance as over one year since last check	Nil	Health and safety training. Ask staff if any have an interest in training in this area to advise the practice
The practice has a policy to ensure the prevention of fraud	No policy but good practice	Practice manager and partner B	Partner B	Write policy	Understanding of the risks and common pitfalls	Discuss with practice accountant and produce written policy
The practice has a protocol for the identification and referral to social services of carers	No	Practice manager	Salaried doctor E	Jointly write policy	Understanding of social services systems to receive information	Write to social services to find out their systems and write and agree policy
There is a written procedure manual that includes staff employment policies	No policy for sick leave or harassment	Practice manager	Partner A	Jointly write policy	Practice manager and partner A to understand issues and write policies	Practice manager and partner A to attend training on employment practice

* Assumes the practice management structure in Box 11.3.

A worked example of creating a practice and personal development plan

The practice has to work through all the quality criteria in the contract and several more. In the example the practice management organisational criteria have been used. For each criterion an action is required. Some are managerial, like the production of a practice protocol, and others are educational, like the learning of a new skill or reference to a knowledge base for an answer.

The practice plan uses the partnership responsibilities set out for the example in Box 11.3. The resulting educational requirements are shown. The areas of responsibility and training for doctor A are shown separately along with the resulting training need (*see* Tables 15.2 and 15.3).

This will not be the only training need for this doctor. All of the requirements are priorities and need to be accomplished this year. As the doctor is going to have a continuing responsibility in this area, investing in a substantial amount of training is appropriate. This could have been done for any of the doctors or the practice manager.

Table 15.3   Part of the personal development plan for doctor A developed from the practice professional development plan.

Organisational standard	Training/course required?	Training required this year	Practice time to be made available
Recording of hepatitis B status and immunisation of clinicians	Private study by partner and contacting medical defence organisation	Understanding of confidentiality issues Course on employment law and good practice	Two days to attend course
Compliance with national guidelines for instrument sterilisation	Nil		
Person specifications and job descriptions are produced for all advertised vacancies	Practice manager and partner A to attend course on employment law and purchase textbook		
The practice has systems in place to ensure regular and appropriate inspection, calibration, maintenance and replacement of equipment	Health and safety training Ask staff if any have an interest in training in this area to advise the practice		
There is a written procedure manual that includes staff employment policies	Practice manager and partner A to attend training on employment practice		

The work and the training need of the practice manager in the worked example are extensive. Where possible, the work, training and continuing responsibility can be delegated to other members of the practice administration staff or shared with experts outside the practice who are called on for specialist knowledge when required. The competences required of managers have been defined and published as part of the contract documentation.

Some of the training areas for the practice staff will require the doctors or other staff to teach. It is entirely appropriate that skills learned are shared with other members of the practice and outside the practice.

The format of the worked example has been chosen to mirror the criteria in the organisational domain but the training could subsequently be modified and divided between the areas of the appraisal framework.

How and when will this occur?

It will take several hours to go through all the relevant criteria and decide the training that is required. It requires a meeting with all of those involved and the practice managerial staff. If clinical criteria are to be discussed, the meeting is likely to involve the partners, salaried doctors, nurses, practice manager and computer staff and possibly more staff. In a large practice it may be necessary to limit the numbers. The meeting will require protected time.

For the organisational tasks discussion may only require the partners and managers. However, if it is likely that tasks will be delegated to staff not present, it is better to involve them.

Box 15.2   An example of a practice clinical meeting

All the practice medical and nursing staff are invited to an education half day and paid whether working at that time or not. The practice's work is looked after by locums.

Half the time is spent going through the clinical criteria and considering the resulting training needs. The remainder of the session consists of individual reports or presentations on the previous personal development plans and the clinical knowledge gained.

Two sessions of paid personal study time are allowed for each participant before the next session to investigate the topic and produce a report for the other clinical members of the practice team.

This process could occur three times a year, avoiding the summer holidays. Other meetings would be required with the administration staff for some or all of the clinical members of the team to understand and co-ordinate their educational activity.

Once the practice has achieved most or all of the education tasks it will need to maintain its good practice. This task is smaller but medicine changes and further training will be required.

Chapter 16

Good practice with medicines

Medicines have become a basic tool in treating illness. Practices hold the repeat prescribing record for all patients and most medicines so the potential for improving patient symptoms and longevity is considerable. If it is established that medicines should be given in certain circumstances then systems should be in place to review whether this is happening or record why it is not happening. Conversely, there is the possibility of incorrect prescribing, inadequate monitoring and drug interactions. This can be reduced by attention to detail when medicines are prescribed and at regular review.

What is expected from the practice?

The principal requirements are to prescribe certain medicines for particular diseases and to review medicines. The guidance is not restrictive and the review can be carried out in person or by telephone, by a doctor or other clinician. Nurses and pharmacists are specifically mentioned.

   The storage of medicines in the practice is important both to maintain the quality of the product and to provide a record of what happens to medicines. This is particularly important for controlled drugs. The acute problems of allergy and immediate reactions to injected medicines are important and the practice needs to be able to respond appropriately. As an example, to show the ability to cope with these requirements, the storage conditions and fridge temperature recordings for vaccines are measured. The batch number and arrangements for resuscitation are also reviewed. A comprehensive list of how the quality of medicine management is assessed is given in Table 16.1.

Table 16.1   How the indicators assess medicine management.

Organisational area	Development need	Organisational standards*	Clinical standards	Patient questionnaire
Prescribing	Recording and appropriate use of prescribing with monitoring for side effects	Presence of record of drugs. Formulary acceptance, repeat prescription availability, some batch no. and expiry date recording, group directions for non-doctors Discussion and review of prescribing with advisor	Use of certain drugs in specific clinical areas	Asks about explanations given to the patient
Medication review	Presence of a contact to check appropriate, monitor and remove redundant prescribing Interactions and side effect monitoring	Presence of a medicine review	Detailed review of illnesses associated with medicines and requirement to prescribe for certain illnesses Monitoring of lithium and patient compliance with antipsychotic drugs	Asks about explanations given to the patient
Medicines storage	Storing medicines in a safe environment Appropriate and recorded use of controlled drugs	Vaccine storage arrangements Adherence to the Medicines Act for storage of controlled drugs and monitoring	Not examined	Not examined
Repeat prescription availability	Efficient and convenient systems to check and make repeat prescriptions available	Repeat prescriptions should be available in 48–72 hours	Not examined but the availability of the system will affect the outcome of chronic disease management	Patient views of the practice and receptionists are affected by the repeat prescription system

* In organisational domain, contractual and statutory requirements and additional services.

Medicine and disease reviews

When the practice is managing chronic diseases uniformly and to a high standard they require review at defined intervals. This can be done by disease or all together on one review. Medicines also require regular review. Most GP computer systems will produce a reminder when the patient has not had a medicine review for a set length of time. It would seem sensible to bring these two review processes together.

This can be done in individual disease management clinics provided the protocol also lists the requirements to review medications. There is considerable overlap between the cardiovascular and diabetes criteria and therefore these could be managed together. This is not true of mental health or thyroid disease.

Regular patient reviews of patients on medication

- Diseases need review
- Several can be reviewed at one time
- Medicine reviews provide an opportunity to review diseases as well as medicines
- Summaries can be updated
- Diseases outside the clinical framework can also be reviewed

---

The amount of GP time is limited at present and practices should make the best use of what is available. One method of doing this is to use the breadth of GP skills to handle acute medical problems at the same time as reviewing chronic conditions and updating disease registers. Most chronic diseases requiring management also require drug therapy. Diseases could be managed by reviewing medication every six months and treating and reviewing the diseases at the same time. This has the advantage of reviewing all illnesses and not just those specified in the clinical domain.

Box 16.1 Utilising a pharmacist for medicine reviews

A practice decided to delegate some medicine reviews to a pharmacist. The pharmacist brought the skills of medicines management and interactions. Training was given in routine monitoring of the common medications. Training was also given in the measurement of blood pressure and the reasons for referring a patient to the doctor if problems were developing.

The annual medication reviews of patients were booked with the pharmacist. Patients were seen and the medication reviewed. Some simple disease reviews involving the measurement of blood pressure were also undertaken. For single diseases medication was changed under a patient group direction. Where multiple diseases were involved changes were made after discussion with doctors.

Reviewing patients on treatment, finding out why the medicine was started and updating the summary list at that time can achieve several tasks required on one appointment. It is time consuming and longer appointments are required both for gathering the data and entering them in a record, presumably the computer. Patient time is also important. Individual pieces of information will be forgotten, blood tests will be missed or not cover all the tests required. Patients will be recalled time and again to get the data required. Anything that reduces the number of times patients have to be called and recalled will save the GPs and patients time.

Box 16.2   An example of a mixed system of GP and nurse review of CHD

The practice decides that it would like to set up a coronary heart disease (CHD) clinic utilising nursing staff. The clinic description and the work to be carried out were originally agreed between the practice and the staff. The description was written by the staff and training arranged.

Patients are invited to attend the clinic by letter generated from the disease index. The invite includes a form for a blood test for renal function, full blood count and cholesterol.

On each clinic appointment the control of any existing symptoms is discussed. The blood pressure, cholesterol, smoking status and influenza and pneumococcal vaccine status are ascertained. The use of a beta-blocker and ACE inhibitor or a contraindication against them is checked against the prescribing record.

Lifestyle advice is given.

If the disease, blood pressure and blood test results show control the medication record is updated and the patient invited to re-attend the clinic in one year. If not, some medicines are altered in the clinic under a patient group direction or referred to the doctor.

If medicines are reviewed annually and the reason for prescribing is entered as a diagnosis, a disease index will be created for many diseases. At the medicine review inappropriate or redundant medication can be stopped and interactions reviewed. Some specific medications require blood monitoring, e.g. lithium. As each medication relates to a disease then the monitoring for those diseases can also be done at the same time. The medicines can be reviewed and updated for a specific length of time and a note made of each disease that has been reviewed. Any information that is required can be entered on an appropriate template as part of the disease review. This is a considerable piece of work and requires a long consultation. However, disease indexes, recording of multiple parameters and outcome measures will rapidly improve. It is also likely to considerably improve the care of individual patients if there are deficiencies.

What should happen at a medicine review?

All repeat medicines should be started for a reason. Checking them against the indication will result in some being stopped and others changed to more appropriate medications. Sometimes a contraindication will be found by reviewing old diagnoses. For example, the patient is on a non-steroidal anti-inflammatory drug (NSAID) and there is an old diagnosis of duodenal ulcer. Summaries produced by the traditional method also miss out some illnesses because of the way they are recorded in GP notes. Osteoarthritis leads to a lot of prescribing that starts with a prescription here or there and then becomes chronic, without formal diagnosis. Reviewing hospital letters or consultations will not show that it is the most important problem for the patient.

Diseases change over time and medication may need to increase or decrease. For example, the blood pressure may have risen or fallen substantially, leading to a change of medication. Interactions can arise as medicines are added. Of course, they shouldn't happen at all but a review of all medicine at one time provides the opportunity to check. The tendency to endorse advice from many different specialists can produce conflict between medicines and the generalist is in a good position to decide between competing priorities.

Some medicines require regular review. The person reviewing the medicines has to know how often blood levels should be monitored and whether any other checks are required, such as regular full blood count, renal or liver function tests.

Tasks for medicine reviews

- Check all medication has a matching problem or disease
- Review care of the diseases
- Review medication still being taken at the appropriate dose
- Check for drug interactions
- Monitoring for drug side effects or problems (blood tests, etc.)

The personnel to carry out the review have not been defined. It could be a nurse in a single disease clinic or a pharmacist looking at the prescribing issues. It could also be the GP. Three different solutions have been described: either the doctor reviews the illness and the medication, the pharmacist provides the medication review and looks at the diseases or the nurse sees the patient in the clinic and patients do not see the doctor. It is for the practice to decide who is most likely to be able to get the patient to attend, who is most likely to record the data and to achieve control of the disease. This may vary from time to time or between practices. The solution arrived at will profoundly affect the job role of the staff. There is a difference between helping the doctor with workload and replacing the doctor. This has implications for the relative number of each type of clinician required and the variety and interest of each job.

Box 16.3 A practice system for reviewing multiple diseases and medicines

A practice wants regular reviews of all medicines and all diseases but wishes to share the workload with nursing staff. Disease management clinics were set up for the common illnesses requiring medication and review (CHD, diabetes, stroke, COPD and asthma). The default review period for medicines is set at six months on the computer. Patients are sent a form for a blood test and an appointment to review their medicines in a clinic after six months before their regular six-monthly review. When they are seen in clinic the computer is reset and a further six months of medication authorised.

If the patient does not have one of the illnesses seen in a clinic the computer will generate a request to see the doctor. The doctor reviews their illnesses and medication. If they feel a longer review interval is required, say a year (for controlled epilepsy or thyroid disease), the review interval is manually altered. If the doctor feels regular blood tests are required at a later date the patient can be given a form or a diary entry made to alert the staff when the next set of regular blood forms should be generated.

This system is used for review of chronic mental health problems but the intervening appointment is with a practice-based community psychiatric nurse (CPN) rather than the practice nurse.

Where patients have multiple illnesses or uncontrolled illness at the nurse clinic, appointments are made with the doctor. In this way continuity and doctor review of multiple illnesses is provided on an annual basis. A significant proportion of the work is delegated. The doctors continue to see patients with a diverse range of illnesses and the blood tests required will have been done before they are seen to allow efficient consultations. The doctors have personal knowledge of the care patients are receiving and complex review arrangements for quality of the nurses' work are avoided.

In addition a practice-based pharmacist conducts some annual reviews of patients on multiple medications to check for interactions.

Chapter 17

Involving patients

What can patients expect from the practice?

Practices are expected to provide services for patients for 45 hours during the week, from Monday to Friday between 8 a.m. and 6.30 p.m. They can open after these hours if they wish. Practices are expected to describe the services offered in a practice leaflet and run an in-house complaints system. The practice will survey patients about their views of services and make changes.

The questionnaires ask about opening hours, whether appointments are easily available, length of wait to appointment and satisfaction with the consultation. This will give a picture of how patients view the service.

The clinical criteria require change from patients. They need to agree to attend appointments, have measurements and blood tests taken and take medication. For some diseases, for instance diabetes, they have to change their lifestyle. This will be difficult and demand trust on the part of the patient. The ability of the GP to see a patient once and review several illnesses and target investigations will be important. The continuity and ongoing relationship with individuals will be important in persuading patients to attend. Even though the control of chronic disease is in their interest, their compliance cannot be taken for granted.

Similarly there is a requirement to measure smoking prevalence and blood pressure across the whole population over 45 years of age. This can be done when attending for other purposes. Creative solutions to encouraging patients to attend will be required.

Table 17.1 How the indicators assess communication with patients.

Organisational area	Development need	Organisational standards*	Clinical standards	Patient questionnaire
Opening hours and contact arrangements	Facilitating easy contact arrangements, appointment and telephone access	Description of contact arrangements and opening hours	Not measured	Specific questions on function
Relationships with patients	Respect and continuity, explanations, personal advice	Complaints system	Requires continuity and excellent relationships to persuade the patient to attend and re-attend for review	Directly questioned
Confidentiality	Holding data confidentially and informing patients about use	Caldecott guardian and the display of a notice	Not examined	Not examined

* In organisational domain, contractual and statutory requirements and additional services.

Encouraging patient contact

It is often assumed that the cause of poor healthcare rests with health professionals and that deficiencies occur because services are not provided. In reality, patients vary considerably in their desire to use medical services. It is known that the educated get much more from the health service and live longer. This effect is not strictly related to wealth but broadly follows education. This is an unacceptable state of affairs and all groups should have good healthcare. It does, however, take more effort and staff time to encourage the whole of the practice population to participate in healthcare and chronic disease management. Patients sometimes find it easier not to attend or do not get onto lists or registers and consequently are not treated. These are the patients who do not receive the best of healthcare. The requirement to measure outcomes across whole populations means that the practice must try to include hard-to-reach groups and improve care.

Encouraging participation from patients who don't normally attend will be important. Practices have shown ingenuity in the past in improving the take-up of smears. Targets set as single levels that attracted payment have been abolished for all clinical criteria. If patients understand what is on offer and decide they don't want it, they can dissent from treatment.

No one knows how important the reputation of the practice and continuity are in encouraging patients to attend. The flexibility and breadth of general practice have traditionally been a strength. If a patient attends for one purpose, usually an acute event, a request for an answer to a question or a specific worry, then, if appropriate, basic health data or specific health data relating to a particular illness, such as blood pressure or cholesterol, can be measured at the same time. This ability to vary the consultation and, within limits, meet the doctor's as well as the patient's agenda is important. It is not known where the limit lies and how many times the patient will be willing to attend surgeries to control illness.

This too will have to be considered in the design of chronic disease management services in the future. Practices cannot assume that because they change their systems and invite patients to participate in care, they will necessarily come.

Educating patients and the expert patient scheme

One way of encouraging patients to receive more care is to inform them about the disease and its management. Patient education programmes have been available for many years. All consultations would expect to provide information about the illness and the additional time available to nurses in existing disease management clinics includes patient education. If some of the diseases in the clinical framework are to be controlled to the highest levels there is a need to change patient lifestyles. This is particularly true of diabetes but there are other diseases where this applies. Information, education and motivation are all required.

Experience elsewhere suggests that patients can understand the issues well and help to educate others. This led to the creation of the expert patient scheme where individual patients are encouraged to learn more and to speak to others about specific illnesses. In time there is the possibility of creating specific literature and other materials to help with explanations of the reasons for treating diseases. This will help practices to convince patients to change their lifestyle and lead to an improvement in the care of disease. PCOs will be expected to provide resources and set up expert patient groups to help practices.

This will not be the only source of patient-written or patient-friendly information but it should prove helpful in dealing with this task.

Encouraging change from patients

- Patients will need to be encouraged to attend for care
- Difficult lifestyle change will be required from them
- Personal relationships will be important
- Patient acceptance of multiple visits to a practice timetable is not guaranteed
- Hard-to-reach groups will have to be included

Obtaining feedback from practice patients

The patient experience requires the practice to consult patients in a specific way. If practices are to meet the requirements of the clinical framework they will need to tailor services to suit all patients. Obtaining information from local patients about their views and how to improve the service is an important method of achieving quality and will also help to encourage patients to attend and improve management of their illnesses.

Two questionnaires have been accepted as valid tools for this purpose. In order to use these tools in a practice setting some thought is required. Valuable information can be obtained about the way the patients view practice services. All surveys of general practice show high personal satisfaction rates and these surveys are likely to follow the same pattern. However, the detail will also help the practice to determine if some services are less well liked or causing some patients difficulty. The practice needs to decide which survey they wish to use and a method of delivery. The questionnaire can be sent by post or given to individuals in the surgery. Someone needs to be available to hand them out, to find writing implements and somewhere to write to help with obtaining completed assessments. There also needs to be somewhere to leave them when they are completed.

Tool 17.1   Issues to be considered in organising a questionnaire survey

Which version of the questionnaire?

Postal and practice versions of the questionnaires are available
The questionnaires work best if the patient has knowledge of consultations

Before the survey

Informing the doctors and nurses that it is to happen
Who will be given the data produced by the questionnaires? Is it private to the individual?
How will administrative staff be informed it is to happen?
How are staff to be involved at different times of day and in branch surgeries?
Fixing a time to give out questionnaires
Is the survey in the surgery or by post?
How are patients to be identified – whole surgeries or random from list?
Is it helpful to co-ordinate with other audits, e.g. advanced access audit?
Is there a patient representative group at the practice? Should they be consulted? Will they want involvement in the design and use of questionnaires?

Getting a good response

1   If distributed in the surgery
    Is a notice in the waiting area required to inform patients it is happening?

Who is going to give the questionnaires out?

How do you identify patients seeing all doctors and nurses in reasonable numbers?

Is there somewhere to sit to fill them out after the consultation?

Are pens and something to write on available?

Is there help available for questions, disadvantaged groups (e.g. visually handicapped)?

Are stamped addressed envelopes to be available if patients want to take questionnaires away?

How is the process to be made confidential?

Does specific staff time need to be made available?

How will staff time be replaced?

Is there a box or other method to collect the completed returns?

2 If distributed by post

How will patients be selected?

Who will write the explanatory letter and what will improve the response rate?

What is the return mechanism? Is a stamped addressed envelope required?

Dealing with the results

How will they be dealt with when they come back to the practice?

Who will analyse them?

How will it be done?

Collating results, e.g. designing spreadsheets to analyse

How will feedback to staff be organised, for individuals and the group?

How will the information be used to change services in the practice?

Who will the result be discussed with as a patient representative?

How are the patients to be informed of the result?

There are national norms available for both tools. There is an additional financial reward when the results are shared and discussed with patient representatives or a PCO appointee. If the practice has understood the results this is likely to be an opportunity to plan new services that suit the needs of the practice population. At present the requests made by PCOs for changes in services are based on the views of the 'average patient'. The contract gives the opportunity to make services appropriate for local needs. This may result in the creation of new models of care, for example services during daylight hours for the elderly. Alternatively, involving patients or patient representatives may lead to greater understanding and a real consideration by patients of the stresses on the service.

How should the practice consult patients?

There are many ways to consult patients or find representatives. The patient participation group is a recognised way of selecting patients to enter into discussion with the practice on behalf of others. Other methods would also be viable. The practice has an alternative of discussing the results of the patient surveys and consultation with a representative of the PCO.

General practice has the largest throughput of any service in the country. It therefore has the opportunity to consult widely and get beyond special interest groups.

Involving patients and senior PCO representatives will help to bring the collective view of patients to a wider audience and produce change outside primary care. Some GPs have said that existing requests for service changes in the name of patients are not helpful to local populations. The patient experience provides encouragement to test that.

In time it is expected that confidence and skills will increase, allowing consultation about complex issues. At present service provision and the site where services are delivered are largely decided by the PCOs as the representative of patients. Many GPs feel that patients would like a different configuration with greater investment in general practice and primary care. Diagnostic facilities and enhanced services could be provided in the community. The tools, patient base and skills will soon exist in general practice to consult patients directly about their views.

Chapter 18

Premises

The requirement to perform more work to a higher standard and to delegate as much of that work as possible to others has been described, as has the need to have managerial facilities in place locally to control and organise that expanded workforce. That workforce needs places to meet and space for education and training. A large proportion of this activity will occur in the premises of the practice. GPs with a special interest (GPwSI) and enhanced services will also need a base to operate from.

This suggests a requirement for improved practice premises of a larger size. New legal requirements specify that disabled access must be provided for staff as well as patients. The contractual and statutory requirements specify minimum levels of provision; they do not describe the specific requirements of property for more developed practices. Premises improvement will need to be planned early because the lead times to build are longer than the time taken to employ staff. They are also complex projects demanding thought and time.

Table 18.1 How the indicators influence use of premises.

Organisational area	Development need	Organisational standards*	Clinical standards	Patient questionnaire
Premises	Multiple expansions to make fit for purpose as practice ascends quality ladder	Physical check on premises to baseline requirements	Larger premises have to be present to house all the staff	Are they comfortable and functional?

*In organisational domain, contractual and statutory requirements and additional services.

Changing requirement for premises with levels of achievement

The concept of base, improving and steady-state practices provides a basis for thinking about premises improvement. It takes time to employ and train staff and build the layers of facilities to improve a practice. Therefore property has to be built and later upgraded. Very large premises could be built initially but too rapid an expansion of staff numbers produces risks. Leaving parts of a building empty until the practice grows into the new facility also has problems and underuses resources.

Therefore flexibility of design and financing to allow later change is required. This is a potential problem for private finance initiative (PFI) schemes where the initial contract can be specified and tendered for competitively but upgrades only have one possible provider and where contract negotiations for unexpected changes are expensive. Medicine and primary care have developed in unexpected directions and even low-tech buildings like GP surgeries rapidly become out of date and require change. There is a need to build into a contract the ability to change the building at a later date if required.

Premises requirements

- Premises will need to expand as the practice ascends the levels of the framework
- This will probably require several modest increases
- Function and internal structure also need to change
- Flexible finance and contracts will be required

Sharing with other professionals and organisations

There is great benefit in networking with other professions within and outside medicine. However, as the size and complexity of surgeries grow the ability to co-ordinate declines as the need for it increases. Placing different groups of professionals in the same building allows this to happen up to a point where the building is so large that socialisation takes place within rather than between staff groups. Where possible the building design should facilitate daily social contact between professions.

GPwSI and consultant chambers

These services are available for an area. It may or may not be appropriate to place them with GPs. Patients can be consulted about their preferences through the practice surveys and patient representatives. This will be dependent on rates of car ownership, transport links and parking.

Funding sources: PCO, LIFT and GP ownership

There are a multitude of possible owners for a building. These could be within the current local improvement finance trust (LIFT) scheme where finance is made available to create and pay rent on premises. LIFT is not currently available everywhere. Premises could be owned and leased back by another business, possibly medically related, like a local or national pharmacy or even a supermarket. Conversely GPs could continue to own and run their own space or a larger building on a rental basis.

The finance all comes from the PCO. They have a budget and discretion to spend it to provide facilities. The current system has many problems. Regular upward-only rent reviews work well in town centres where property appreciates in rental and value. The initial difficulty in finding sites is overcome by flexibilities to purchase land quickly. PCOs have more discretion about payment methods and options to help practices create viable developments away from areas where property automatically appreciates in value. Practices can elect to have rental increases in line with inflation and PCOs can provide stability for the owners by their flexibility to continue the lease if the practice no longer wishes to continue ownership.

Chapter 19

Why does the practice need a business plan?

The practice needs to organise itself and provide an environment that allows clinicians to treat the patients. It needs to be managed sufficiently to allow this to happen. The business plan is a method of describing and co-ordinating the different functional areas of the practice (e.g. IT, staff, training) and explaining this to others. Many of the areas of a non-NHS business plan do not apply. The vision of the business, market and payment structures are all given and do not need to be repeated unless work outside the NHS is anticipated.

What management is required?

The partners have a contract on behalf of the practice with the PCO. They are ultimately personally responsible for the level of service provided by the practice. They employ staff and have systems to achieve tasks. There needs to be a method for them to understand how they are going to achieve that and to enable the partners to describe this to the PCO and the practice.

The indicators in the contract provide a method of demonstrating high-quality care although they are not comprehensive. The management functions listed in Table 19.1 provide a series of tools to help the practice to manage itself.

Table 19.1   How the indicators assess practice management.

Organisational area	Development need	Organisational standards*	Clinical standards	Patient questionnaire
Practice policies	Locally appropriate methods of dealing with administrative tasks that work, are known to staff and patients alike	Request to write policies and discuss with PCO. Check on implementation at practice visit	Audit policies, data handling, generation of letters, call and recall must be present to achieve the standards	Patient acceptance of policies often described in answer to questions on relationships with staff
Business planning	Ability to understand environment and plan for future	Requirement to involve staff in the business plan	Ability to self-organise to succeed; requires self-review and PDSA cycles	Indirectly in quality of service and directly with small group or by survey for specific purposes
Learning from experience/risk management	Constant improvement to a learning organisation	Significant event audit	Change in organisation required to achieve clinical standards Managing chronic illness reduces risk of premature death	Not examined
Health and Safety	Use of appropriate equipment in a safe environment for staff and patients	General requirement and specific task monitoring, equipment monitoring	Not examined	Not examined
Financial integrity	Protection from fraud or non-payment of wages	Checking on who authorises what payment for staff, not partners. Protection of the partners is a good idea but not specified by the contract	Not examined	Not examined

* In organisational domain, contractual and statutory requirements and additional services.

Creating the business plan

Once a practice has looked at its current performance and decided where it would like to go with IT, staff and training, it will need to co-ordinate change in several different areas at one time. It is not possible to employ staff to work on an IT system that hasn't been installed or train staff that haven't been employed yet. The practice business plan is the place to list the expected changes and present them in such a way as to show how co-ordination will be achieved.

The business plan will list changes by area of interest and the timescales over which change will occur. The limitation on the amount of work that individuals can produce will force the practice to prioritise and co-ordinate training and development. There are limits to how many new staff can be integrated into the practice and how much development can take place in a short time. Decisions need to be taken and all staff members kept informed and motivated to produce change. Doing this well constitutes good management. Those practices that achieve this will perform well.

Content of the business plan

- Summary of expected changes by organisational area
  - IT
  - Practice workforce
  - Practice training
  - Internal system change
  - Premises
- Expected changes with time
- Expected costs
- Expected income
- Co-ordination and phasing of developments as infrastructure develops

---

The partners and manager in the practice need to understand the integration of all the changes expected. That understanding is as important for the practice as the finished document. The finished document is required for the staff and to refer back to as implementation proceeds.

The business plan is also helpful as a source of information to request help from outside the practice. If it is clear the number of staff have to increase then the number of computer terminals will also have to increase. This would provide a powerful argument to approach the PCO and ask for additional resources.

Box 19.1 How expansion in one area of the practice requires change elsewhere

A practice decides to increase its chronic disease management capability. In order to do this it will set up nurse-run clinics. It will limit this to two whole-time equivalent nurses in the first year and diabetes and CHD clinics.

In order to support the nurses it needs two extra computers, use of two rooms and an extra half-time receptionist to make appointments and greet the patients on the day. The receptionist will require the use of a room and computer for two hours per week to make appointments and can use the existing terminal on the desk during the clinic. Some training will be required for the receptionist. Additional throughput of repeat prescriptions will require more time to process and more checking of prescriptions. A doctor will require time to help write the clinic protocols and oversee the clinics. Time will also be required to help with clinical problems encountered in the clinics. Additional work in appraising and managing the new employees can be absorbed. The new staff will require time to attend courses to prepare them for the new role.

The substantial amount of new clinic time results in changes to:

- Nurses' time
- Reception staff
- Room use
- IT equipment
- Doctors' clinical time
- Prescription systems
- Practice professional development plan and cost.

In time the practice facilities that didn't change in this example would also come under strain. Changes would be required to the number of managers, the computer server, telephone system and the premises.

Methods to plan with

The issues that need to be co-ordinated have already been developed in this book. By working through the tools to decide what change is required for each domain and the contractual and statutory requirements a list will be produced. This is likely to be long, as most criteria require some change in IT and staff and training.

In order to plan, the requirements for each functional area of the practice need to be teased out. A series of headings are given but the practice could increase or reduce the number depending on what they are trying to achieve.

Major headings to use for understanding and integrating development

- Staff
  - Partnership tasks
  - Doctor tasks
  - Nurse tasks
  - Management tasks
  - Administration tasks
  - IT tasks
- IT systems
  - Hardware
  - Software
- Practice equipment (telephone, ECG machine, etc.)
- Practice professional development plan
- Premises

Table 19.2 Relating functional areas to development over time for a CHD clinic.

Year	CHD clinic	Planning	Employing staff	IT equipment	Training	Doctor time	Room available for use
2003		Who is required for clinic and initial training need		Audit to show the size of the task and hence the amount of time required to see the patients			
		Writing the clinic protocol with the staff	Employ nurses	Ability to call and recall	Training in CHD for nurses		
2004	Starts operating		Employing new clerk to run clinic	New computers in place	Induction training of the new clerk and specific training on running the clinic	More time to help with teething problems and day-to-day issues	Rooms required
	Operating					Patients with partially controlled disease now referred to doctors for action	Rooms required
2005	All patients now seen for annual check				Audit of clinic effectiveness and of the change produced	Lower input as most patients now controlled	
	Operating	Review of effectiveness			Nurses report to doctors on effect of clinic		

For each heading the plan needs to show development over time to demonstrate the implications of a plan and the order in which change has to happen.

The example shows how staff have to be employed and trained before the clinic starts and how other staff members can be employed later and will have to be trained in the ways of the practice as much as in the specific job role required. The IT requirements come in three phases: finding out the size of the task at the planning stage, calling and recalling patients as the clinic starts and auditing success. Different people may do each IT task. The initial audit could be done by the practice manager, the call and recall by the newly employed clerk and the final audit by the clinicians who run the clinic.

It is entirely possible to draw lines for each area representing time and add the significant changes freehand. This process can be done for a larger number of changes. The list of changes required to meet the criteria of the contract can be divided between the different functional areas. The amount of change required in each functional area will be large. It is not possible to do everything in one or two years and practices will need to plan over several years to achieve the changes required.

It will be obvious that some actions are not possible because the staff or premises infrastructure are not there to support the changes. This is a valuable insight for the practice. The practice can work out when the new premises or support staff are required and look at the length of time taken to train or build a solution. This often requires attention to property and infrastructure as one of the first changes.

Box 19.2   Planning for premises

Planning for premises should be done early.

Premises easily become the limiting factor in development. As practices develop and doctors devolve clinical work to others, the length of time with the patient increases. Support for the clinic requires the doctor to be available even if doing something else. The doctors' appointments are also lengthened. Administering the practice systems takes more time, usually in meetings or on the computer in a surgery room. Teaching and training increase. Taking additional attached staff into the practice also uses rooms. At low interest rates the financing costs on a £1 million building are less than the cost of one salaried doctor. It is worth planning early for premises and having some spare capacity.

Who is going to do the planning?

The partnership will need to decide where the management roles outlined as competences in the contract are to be provided. If partners are to provide the strategic leadership for the business then the tasks and areas of development will have to be apportioned as areas of responsibility. If the practice manager is to have that role then this will need to be discussed and agreed.

Planning for the practice takes time and focus. The practice has to decide who is doing the planning and involve a moderate number of people, probably including the partners but maybe also the practice manager and some key employed staff or clinicians. The top team needs time away from the everyday job to discuss the strategic issues and develop solutions. As a practice starts to develop from base level, the complexity of the co-ordination required is manageable and can be organised by meetings scheduled into the working day. As the practice becomes more complex and employs more people, some time away from the practice is likely to be required so the partners will have to reduce their commitment to clinical work. If the practice tries to do it as an extra, by the time it has become a large and complex organisation the workload will be too much for most people.

Box 19.3 Meeting schedule for a large developed practice

Partnership meetings

Monthly business meeting – two hours
Weekly business meetings – simple problems and to pass information
Annual strategy meetings – to plan for major changes: two meetings of
   three hours

Co-ordination meetings

Three-monthly with representatives of employed and attached staff
Three-monthly with employed doctors
Ad hoc additional meetings related to new developments

Education meetings

Three-monthly PPDP meetings to set future agenda and report on
   personal study
Meetings within staff groups for training and development of each other
Time for personal study outside meetings

A hybrid system is more likely and some strategic roles may not be within the competence of the individuals within the practice. It may be appropriate to seek help from PCO managers, for strategic issues involving more than one practice, or from a management consultancy. The quality criteria can be achieved with internal management resources. Over time experience of outside managers should be used to improve skills and develop internal capacity. The process then becomes developmental for the practice and the individuals within it.

It is possible that some practices will not feel confident enough to develop business plans of their own in the first few years of the contract. Most practices should have the ability but may not have the experience. A business plan requires a list of tasks to be accomplished in different areas and a method of inter-relating the changes in one area to another over time. It is possible to have help with this writing process using an external resource. The practice should aim to use their own ideas and methods to learn how to create a plan for the future.

Planning outside the practice

The business plan will also need to identify gaps and problems outside the practice that will impede success with the contract. For example, left ventricular dysfunction cannot be diagnosed by echocardiography if there is inadequate capacity for GPs to use. It will be necessary to work with the PCO to achieve change. Provision and quality of secondary care are likely to variable so part of the task will be to identify those changes and encourage solutions. The initiative of GPs with a special interest provides an alternative way of achieving specific tasks.

Influencing care outside the practice

- Gap analysis (areas where external services not available or not performing)
- Bringing problems to the attention of the PCO
- Joint planning of solutions
  - Enhanced services
  - GPwSI services
  - Change in other services

Implementing the business plan

Once the plan is written it then becomes a matter of administration to implement change according to a timetable. Individual tasks are divided up and allocated. Regular reviews of each area will give an overview of progress towards the whole plan. Some areas will be achieved and others will be more difficult. The business plan has to be kept under constant review to keep development co-ordinated and ensure that all the staff are employed running services at a high level of efficiency.

The method suggested for developing the business plan, of working through the criteria and allocating tasks to an individual, will produce clarity of responsibility. The allocation of the tasks to different people could result in no action because they do not work together. Success with planning requires the individuals in the practice to co-operate. Practices are still going to be small organisations so it should be possible to co-ordinate activity and have good interpersonal contact. Incentives (improving patient care, pride in achievement, autonomy and resources for achieving the criteria) should be used by partners attempting to persuade staff to change.

Chapter 20

Managing the money

The contract does not specify which staff should be employed or reimburse staff salaries. There is no designated amount per GP or regulated number of staff per population. There is no requirement to apply to an external body to increase or reduce the number of GPs, nurses or administrative staff. The contract sum remains the same however many staff are employed.

Investing for greater gain

As the practice improves performance on the Quality and Outcomes Framework it will receive increased funding to pay more staff. Part of the funding should be regarded as a resource for the practice and not all as GP income. The costs of the additional staff are offset against the increased resources that come to the practice. The payments for achieving quality are sufficiently large to cover the additional investment costs and allow substantial gain. Even if the practice is not efficient in its planning, income will still go up and costs be covered. In time the practice can revise staff structures to improve efficiency. Payments are made before staff are employed (aspiration payments) to allow that development to take place.

The business plan should help the practice understand what is happening with its income. The practice will have a list of the number of staff and the training required for any development. It can also estimate the increase in achievement of particular criteria. Both the increased cost and increased income can be calculated. This will be approximate but should give valuable information.

The contract provides resources and the aspiration payment is made to allow staff and facilities to be in place to achieve change later. The practice has to manage the cash available to do this. Therefore if, for example, the practice decides it needs to employ an additional computer clerk to enter data present in the paper notes, it will need to achieve that new task to get the additional income (achievement payment).

Development plans will have to be robust and costed or the practice will be paying for the new staff without receiving the achievement payment. Until now GMS practices have received payments separately from achievement. Planning will become more important in the new environment. Once again autonomy comes with the price of self-organisation and achievement.

The global sum is not intended to be all salary

The contract documentation clearly states that the amount of money entering practice will increase by 31% from 6.1 to 8 billion pounds. If that money does not come into practices there is a mechanism to check and change the payments to reach that amount. If the payment structure does not achieve that there is a guarantee to change it.

As the total amount coming to practices is increasing by 31% there will be an increase for GP salary and practice costs, including staff and training. Practices are already paying substantial sums to staff and increasing that leaves considerable space to employ more staff at improved rates of pay. Practices are already responsible for the costs of training their staff. The money for IT and premises has been allocated separately but is also increased. If all the extra money went into GP income it would rise by more than 31%.

There will be additional costs. More staff and more training will be required. Allocating the global sum to the practice enables it to control the workforce and use the resources of the practice efficiently. GPs have shown themselves adept at this in the past. The money for training and staff should be used wisely. It is possible to increase spending in all areas and still produce a substantial rise in GP income.

Practices already receive payments to employ staff. These are now within the global sum. Practices that already have high staff budgets will have the cost covered through the minimum practice income guarantee (MPIG). They will have less requirement to increase investment. Practices that currently do not employ many staff will have an increase in their funding through the global sum. The new staff can be employed from this sum and the additional resource from quality payments will be income.

Financial efficiency

The increase of 31% on staff funding will go to paying more staff under the government initiative *Agenda for Change*. If the cost of staff members increases faster than GP income it will be financially appropriate to reduce delegation. If GPs become relatively more costly then greater delegation is favoured. Clinical staff, particularly GPs and nurse practitioners, are in short supply so their incomes are likely to rise. The most efficient strategy is to maximise delegation to clerical staff and utilise doctors and nurses for clinical tasks.

Some practices already employ sufficient staff to achieve the criteria of the contract. These developed practices are already receiving substantial staff payments and their ability to increase the global income of the practice will be less but their additional investment to achieve the criteria will also be less. This is also true of PMS practices which have had resources to invest in staff.

Practices with few staff and a long way to go to achieve quality have a lot of leeway to increase their spending as their resources will increase by large amounts. Planning may be a problem as they are less developed but even crude calculations will show that increasing achievement of criteria will bring substantial additional resources.

Cash flow

It was demonstrated in the chapter on business planning that investment in staff and training comes before seeing the patients with a chronic illness and achieving control of the illness. There can be a considerable lag time before investment pays off. The practice can use the aspiration payment to employ and train staff. The achievement payment will arrive in the following year. Therefore practices need to be careful and take time to develop. It would be a major step to build new premises, double the number of staff, introduce new systems and manage all those new people. It can be done but the practices most in need are likely to have the weakest management ability. They will need help with planning but would also benefit from employing a competent manager.

Box 20.1   Cash flow challenges in investing in new clinics

Cash flow in investment decisions for diabetes and CHD clinic

Aim of project: to increase diabetes points from 20 to 70 and CHD from 20 to 80 over two years.
Practice size: 5500 patients.
Costs:
- 2003 Employing 0.33 wte practice nurse for 3 months (£2500). Training (£500)
- 2004 Salary and on cost (£10 000)
- 2005 Salary and on cost (£10 000)

Resources

- 2003 (No assessment of points) Preparation payment £9000. Total £9000
- 2004 (Start of year 40 points) Preparation payment £3250 and aspiration payment £75 × 100 × a third = £2500. Achievement payment £75 × 100 × two thirds = £5000. Total £10 750
- 2005 (Start of year 100 points) Preparation payment £3250 and aspiration payment £120 × 150 × a third = £6000. Achievement payment 120 × 150 × two thirds = £12 000. Total £21 250
- 2006 (Start of year 150 points)

In reality the income in 2004 would be increased by other contract provisions or would be protected by the MPIG.

The existing spending on nurses is included in the current income of practices and it may be that this cost could be met out of the baseline (global sum) funding.

GMS practices will also have an extra income stream. As GMS payments increase before the contract starts, their income will start to rise. This will give opportunities to invest for greater gain later in addition to smaller but significant increases in the first year. When GMS finishes in 2004 there will be a considerable number of item-of-service fees in the system. Maternity, contraception, minor operations and some other fees are paid in arrears. The new payments will start straight away. This is not really additional income but it does provide an additional cash sum to invest in staff for later increases in income. PMS practices have already had this sum of money.

Two criteria have been treated differently in the contract due to the high cost and potential cash flow problems involved. These are the criteria for patient access and summaries in the Quality and Outcomes Framework. If they are not already being achieved they are likely to be expensive to change. They are also true targets as payments only arise when set levels are achieved. Similar directed enhanced services have been created to fund progress towards achievement of the criteria. In this way the cash flow risk of investing in summarisation and the one-off increase in appointments to reduce waiting times can be funded.

Practices are in a better position to invest than normal businesses. The payments for quality are not cash limited. If practices invest and commit to improvement the income will arrive when they are successful. This stability of the market is a major benefit compared to other businesses where the market can disappear after the investment has been made.

Moving beyond personal money to a business that invests

There has been a tendency of practices and partnerships to see themselves as businesses that maximise income and treat investment with caution. If there is no short-term direct payback, investment will not happen. The creation of payments to induce specific actions increases this. These perverse incentives have gone. It is clear what practices should achieve and investment is judged against the likely benefit, clinical and financial.

It is therefore in the practice's interest to make change early and obtain the increased payments. Incomes will rise for the partners when this happens. Practices can only be successful if their staff stay loyal and work for the practice over time. There is additional benefit in continuity for patients if staff stay in the same practice. Practices will need to consider how much the way staff are treated, the fabric of the working environment and the training and development opportunities available to them will affect their willingness to stay.

These wider benefits are obtained by thinking about the business as a whole and improving the working environment and prospects for everyone. Good, well-paid, interesting jobs with autonomy and pride in a job well done are important. Investment in infrastructure and staff support is an important part of making staff feel valued.

This requires thinking about investment over a longer period of time and considering a large number of benefits on the positive side of investment decisions. Allocating money for staff training and meetings is one aspect; another is sufficient equipment and adequate premises to allow flexibility and good use of time.

Investment priorities

- Allocated budget for staff training
- Allocated budget for equipment
- Quality of the working environment, adequate desks and staff rest rooms, etc.
- Paying for staff to attend meetings in practice time, not personal time
- Adequate numbers of staff

Investment decisions

- Including all the costs and benefits of decisions
- Taking a long view of investment payback
- Thinking of some practice money as a resource and not personal income not taken

---

Chapter 21

The role of the primary care organisation

The vision of the contract is a clear statement of what the practice should achieve and allocation of resources to the practice to allow it to do so. The detail of the internal management structure is for the practice to decide. Practices are to be macro-managed, not micro-managed. The consequence of not achieving the quality criteria is a reduced income for the practice.

In giving autonomy to the practice, the levers of change are removed from the PCO. This affects staff finances and incentive schemes. The ability to only give new money if particular staff structures are put in place has gone. In clinical areas the responsibility of practices is clear. A small number of criteria in the organisational and patient experience domains require co-operation with the PCO in agreeing practice objectives. As each criterion is independent, practices will be in a position to decide if the income gained is worth the change requested. This is still a lever albeit a small one.

This was done because the increasing control and management of practices was producing problems. It was not delivering uniform change and it is suggested that it was partly responsible for the recruitment problems in general practice. There is a need for PCOs to recognise this change and manage in a different way. It is possible to achieve more by facilitating and teaching the practices how to manage themselves than by doing it for them. The internal structure and methods of working are different for a facilitative approach to practice managements.

Macro-management of practices

- Clear statement of aims (contract quality criteria)
- Leaving responsibility with practices
- Encouraging local experimentation and solutions (local PDSA cycles)
- Facilitating access to information sources (journals, external guidelines)
- Encouraging revision of external information to produce practice guidelines
- Facilitating peer group support
- Encouraging practices to share methods and solutions
- Managers participating in practice events and teaching management skills
- Helping to solve problems, not imposing external solutions
- Creating local leaders
- Utilising external quality schemes perhaps using the local leaders

PCOs and managers already know that micro-management of practices is difficult and do not necessarily want to do it. However, they have had priorities and targets put into their contracts that were not priorities for GPs. Changing this was one of the reasons for creating the contract.

PCO responsibilities are complementary to practices

The PCO has the responsibility, called a patient guarantee, for ensuring that the service under the new contract is at least as good as the existing service. Where practices have the option of opting out (additional services, some directed enhanced services, out-of-hours services), PCOs have a requirement to provide an alternative service to at least the same standard. If the practice provides the service and succeeds, the PCO responsibility is met. If the practice chooses not to provide it, the PCO has to do so using the same financial resources offered to the practice. PCOs have the resource and a requirement to arrange for all the enhanced services to be provided.

Box 21.1   The PCO responsibility for access to services

The PCO has a requirement to provide access to a primary care practitioner in line with the national requirement. The practice has the option of achieving this target and receiving a payment. If it does not, the PCO has to achieve it using the same amount of money outside the practice.

   It could provide the service by setting up a walk-in clinic or purchase it from another provider for a payment. The practice has an option; the PCO has a responsibility.

In this way a series of overlapping and complementary requirements are made of practices and PCOs. These requirements also apply to the rest of the quality criteria. The PCO has a requirement to create and deliver health improvement plans. The detail will overlap with practice requirements in the Quality and Outcomes Framework. Meeting the requirements of the organisational framework will meet many of the clinical governance requirements of the PCO. Both organisations are required to achieve the same things stated in different ways.

   It is in the interests of the PCO to build capacity, both clinical and managerial, within primary care (GP practices and community services) to meet this challenge. The greater the capacity in these organisations, the less cost in staff time and management focus at the PCO. The PCO has many responsibilities and does not have the time to be involved in day-to-day decisions within external organisations.

   If a skill is required to be successful within the framework then the PCO does not need to have close involvement and control. It has to stimulate the practice to develop and help it on its way when asked. It can monitor success through the Quality and Outcomes Framework and the visiting process.

PCO as commissioner

If direct management and involvement in general practice is not the role of the PCO, what should it be doing? It has a strategic role in running the local health economy. It is expected to understand what is happening across the whole area and how the individual service providers contribute to a cohesive health service that appears seamless to the service user. The commissioning role is a powerful one that allows new services to be shaped.

There is also a role in bringing the individual choices of providers, whether practices or trusts, together to create sufficient demand to commission support services. For example, an individual practice might be too small to organise high-quality postgraduate education but facilitating meetings between practices will stimulate debate and change that is driven by the professional groups themselves. In time, the PCO will be able to withdraw from the service as it becomes self-supporting because of its worth to practices.

All the original responsibilities of the PCO remain, including the requirement to stay in budget despite extreme pressure. It is not helpful to list the other responsibilities as they change rapidly over time and encompass many objectives outside primary care.

PCO commissioning role in primary care

- Responsibility for services to area populations, not practice populations
- Commissioning services to provide a comprehensive whole
- Facilitating joint education and service provision between practices

---

This system works well if practices accept their new responsibilities and work towards achieving them by improving every year. It also assumes that the areas not measured by the Quality and Outcomes Framework continue to be delivered to a high standard. The PCO is accountable for the quality of healthcare provided across the community and will need methods to help practices achieve quality.

Ensuring quality without the traditional levers of change

The PCO has a responsibility to achieve the priorities given to it, usually expressed as targets. For quality targets this is clinical governance, in two areas: helping and encouraging the willing to improve and dealing with unacceptably poor practice.

The seven requirements of CHI will be met if practices achieve the higher levels of the Quality and Outcomes Framework. The development and governance agendas are dependent on practice success. The quality criteria provide the agenda for practices, focusing on the issues included, which encompass most of the priorities given to the PCO. The PCO can map the tasks achieved by the quality framework and the much smaller list of other requirements can then be made known to practices and used as the base for other practice schemes.

The PCO has responsibility for commissioning enhanced services. Some will be national but others will be created locally. The same thinking is relevant to designing these local services. The task should be clearly defined and clinically appropriate. The scheme and its monitoring should provide resources, autonomy and professional pride in a job done well. Each measure should be as near to outcome as possible and criteria and standards developed.

When PCO managers are requesting change or activity they should reflect on what the professionals, including GPs, are likely to feel about that change and what impact it will have on the drivers. This should affect the substance of what is asked and the presentation of the change to practices. There are ways of changing an initiative to fit with the drivers. The detail of how this was done in designing the contract has been described.

The drivers of change for GPs apply.

- Improved patient care
- Professional pride
- Retained autonomy
- Additional financial resources
- Because they were asked to.

PCO managers are likely to be successful if they use these five drivers to produce incentives. GPs will then achieve the PCO managers' targets as part of their normal daily routine.

New levers for change

- Design schemes to achieve improved clinical care
- Work with the values of practitioners
- Create new skills within practices for self-management
- Use the resources of the professions
- Celebrate success to create professional pride

Whilst the quality criteria of the contract are intended to signpost improvement, they will also expose poor performance. Practices that perform poorly or decline to enter the voluntary Quality and Outcomes Framework still have to demonstrate compliance with the contractual and statutory requirements. Improving practices from this low level will be a priority for PCOs. If practices prove incapable then the patient guarantee comes into force and PCOs will provide or commission services.

PCO contacts with the practices

As a minimum all practices will receive an annual assessment. Practices would also benefit from more frequent visits to discuss progress and be reminded of the global task facing them. It is in the practice's and PCO's interest to find out early if progress has stalled and generate solutions.

The management resources of the PCO are required over time to help with the practice planning because the development agenda is large and practices will have to assimilate one round of change before embarking on another. The discussion about next year's development could occur after the assessment visit or at another time. There is a requirement to work with pharmacy advice and the option of discussing the output of the patient questionnaire. These and other contacts with the PCO will go on during the year. The important discussions about IT and premises are managerial, not specialist. The phasing of IT and premises development is part of business planning and broad concepts need to be discussed there. The specialist discussions about building design or which computer hardware to use occur elsewhere.

The practice and PCO will benefit from creating a relationship over time between the same individuals. Those individuals need to have knowledge of available resources to help practices. They therefore have to be senior in the PCO. They will also need to be able to look at the practice work and produce solutions. They will need to know how to accomplish everyday practice tasks or direct them to other resources to provide practical help. They become a helper to the practice and, if requested, assist by commenting on practice plans in production. They can also help by signposting resources and people with other skills to help the practice develop.

The assessment visit is important to practices. It is going to be difficult for the same person to be the judge of so much income and facilitator at the same time. The PCO will have to give careful thought to the composition of the visiting team. There has to be some tension in the role of the local manager. Practices will have to be told to do more on occasion. There is benefit in separating the role of assessor and manager from helper and confidant. With so much money resting on achievement, assessments will have to be rigorous. Professional organisations and peer support provide a mechanism to assist practices outside the management loop.

Tasks for the PCO manager supporting practices

- Avoiding the creation of dependent practices
- Working out the areas and amount of support different practices are likely to require
- Mapping which personnel groups are most likely to be able to provide this support to different levels of practice
- Using the external quality schemes to fill education gaps
- Facilitating interpractice visiting and educational exchange

Use of external and professional resources

Practices are not doing uniformly well at the moment. There is much to do and PCOs have a substantial role in that change but they do not need to do all of it themselves. They can work through external organisations and professional bodies. PCOs have strategic management skills but they are not necessarily experienced in writing policies to get the phone answered or receptionist job descriptions. People currently working in general practice may be better able to help with these.

Generating professional pride requires practices to feel that they have done something that is based on values and has been done well. The professions collectively create a value system and judge whether it has been achieved. It cannot be externally imposed because it would then cease to be a professional value. That is not to say that values cannot change with time or be externally influenced but they have to be changed by debate and, ultimately, agreement.

There is no one organisation within medicine that would be trusted everywhere but there is a need to work with existing representative and professional organisations. Fortunately several organisations have created and continue to work on local tools and support services for change. However, the pressure on GP time, not least in the contract, will reduce the amount that can be given to colleagues for no reward.

The PCO needs a mechanism to find and pay for one or more professionals locally to help others improve. They need to be independent of the PCO and preferably linked to a professional organisation. The professional organisation can then provide quality assurance and the tools. Whilst there are other options (e.g. Health Quality Service), this could mean contracting with the RCGP for several practices to enrol in the QTD or QPA schemes and finding funding or agreeing for the practices to fund a local advisor to help with the process. Practice managers may wish to participate in Fellowship by Assessment of the Institute of Healthcare Management.

Box 21.2 Creating skills for assessment and quality in general practice

Phase 1

Funding for a small number of committed individuals to achieve personal quality schemes, say five per PCO for MAP* or FBA* or FBA**
Encourage practices to complete QTD* or QPA*
Bring together the individuals (doctors, nurses and managers) who complete the assessments to form a peer group

Phase 2

Encourage the peer group to facilitate QPA and QTD across the PCO. Funding for use of the scheme and facilitators falls on PCO. Practice costs are funded by improved performance in Quality and Outcomes Framework

Phase 3

Encourage and fund individuals in all practices to achieve personal quality schemes

* All from the Royal College of General Practitioners
** FBA of the Institute of Healthcare Management

These schemes leave responsibility with the practice. The contract has created the need for the practice to focus its development on this agenda. The PCO can facilitate skills development by bringing in professional organisations respected by the practices themselves.

The contract is dependent on the development of skills in practices. It is expensive and sometimes frustrating to wait for the practices to realise a need and meet it. However, once skills have been gained they can be used and less input is required in future. They can also be used outside the specific areas in the contract. For example, the clinical areas have a wide range but do not include every disease. In time practices can use the skills to examine new areas and can do this without external monitoring. As the quality schemes mentioned are professionally driven they can use formative methods that are not present in the contract. This will bring long-term benefits for practices, patients and the PCO.

In order to provide these support services locally there is a need for training and skills among GPs and other professionals. Investment in training individuals and assisting them to obtain a wide range of qualifications will help the local health community. Practices should fund the standard training but MSc, MD, MBA or FBA of the RCGP probably demand more resources than practices can supply and they benefit the area more than the practice. Funding should come from general PCO resources.

Creating skills in the local health economy

- External organisations already have schemes and tools for this
- Local support is helpful but needs funding for individuals to give the time
- The individuals to give the support and leadership need to be found and trained

---

Specific contract tasks

Review of the criteria in the contract and the variable existing practice abilities detailed earlier suggest that practices will need help and access to resources. There is variability in the number of staff employed by practices, clinical outcomes and the ability to manage strategically.

Managerial support

When a practice improves it has to plan and change working practices. If the practice has not done this before it does not necessarily know what any other practice is doing. Some of those plans will benefit from review by someone else to formatively assess progress and make suggestions. For some areas a manager would be appropriate, for others a clinician. The existing RCGP quality schemes broadly address this need. Whether provided by that route, or another, practices will need feedback about certain areas:

- Management and planning
- Clinical skills
- Personnel management
- Audit and using the data to produce change
- Knowledge of pharmaceutical agents.

Some of these are areas in which the PCO has traditionally been involved. However, help from the PCO will only be used if it meets the need of practices and they choose to be involved.

Holding information

In other areas practices should be able to use existing information and implement change without detailed formative review. The PCO can act as a source for information about how to perform some of the required tasks.

- Instrument decontamination and sterilisation
- Local child protection procedures
- Where and how to refer carers to social services
- How to perform significant event reviews
- PCO receiving the output of significant events and overseeing change in the local health economy
- How to write summaries
- Tools to check and improve the accuracy of disease registers
- Courses for basic life support skills
- Expert patient schemes
- Setting up patient participation groups.

Most of these tasks were previously the responsibility of clinical governance staff.

Gap analysis

The PCO is responsible for commissioning services from secondary care for practices to use. If there is no local service available for the numbers involved, this will be an exclusion. Practices will automatically pass the criterion but patients will not receive the service. The PCO needs to look for the gaps in service provision before the contract is in place and arrange for services to be provided. Therefore it needs to go through each clinical, organisational and patient experience criterion and judge the quality and availability of the service locally. This 'gap analysis' is a major piece of work and a technique applicable in other areas of PCO responsibility.

   As the gaps identified relate to a need in practices and primary care, these gaps represent appropriate areas for enhanced services commissioned from practices in the community with appropriate support. In this way responsibility for the whole of these diseases can be passed to primary care with a new and separately commissioned service not dependent on the needs of secondary care. The advent of GPwSIs will help with this process.

Services likely to be strained by the contract

- Echocardiography for left ventricular failure (LVF)
- Computer tomography (CT) scan for new CVA
- Exercise ECG for angina
- Fundoscopy for diabetics
- Micro-albuminuria testing for diabetics
- Referral for control of epilepsy
- Spirometry for COPD
- Blood testing

Experience in health services across the globe shows that more can be provided for the same budget in the community. The cost saving comes from the whole system, not in individual services. Developing capacity and skills within practices is important.

Currently GPs find it difficult to take time out of practice to attend planning meetings. Erratic attendance makes consultation and service planning difficult. GPwSI schemes provide the opportunity to contract for regular sessional commitments. This will allow time for primary care professionals to attend meetings and design a different kind of service.

Allocation of resources

Specific planning tasks for the PCO

- IT
- Premises
- Enhanced services

As practices take on new tasks they will need bigger premises and more complex IT. Devolving chronic disease management to nurses requires the same number of appointments and longer consultations than with doctors. This will put pressure on the size of the premises in all practices, not just those starting to offer chronic disease management. In order to take on new staff and enhanced services, practices will need space to use. The lead time on development is long so investment and allocation of funding are needed well in advance of practices taking on new initiatives.

Provision will require local planning. The issues are discussed elsewhere but the same principles apply. If the PCO uses its power to enforce IT and premises solutions that diminish the individual practice's ability to control its internal environment then the benefit of autonomy elsewhere in the contract will be lost.

This applies to the computer system provided but the number of systems is likely to reduce and the common standards required may force the systems to look similar. It also applies to the staff and skills to run them. As the systems become more complex there is a tendency for IT professionals above the level of the practice to take over the running of systems, design templates and dominate use of systems. Practices will need help and support from IT professionals but they need to be able to run their own systems and audit their own information. Thus the practice needs high-level skills in entering data and using systems. These skills will need to be duplicated in every practice.

The PCO as provider

The PCO has the freedom to set up its own services within primary care and can create or run its own practices. The contract allows this as part of the freedom to employ practitioners. This can be very positive and alleviate the stress on practices and bring new doctors or other professionals into the labour pool. The PCO also has a responsibility to provide or commission services for patients if practices are unwilling or unable to do this.

If these are autonomous and allocated resources in the same way as other practices, they will soon float free of the PCO. If they are owned and controlled centrally with more resources, they will destabilise practices. This is likely to cause difficulties for GMS practices and ultimately likely to lead to demoralisation. In a competitive environment for GPs between PCOs and a labour shortage, this will not help PCO targets. There is a need for sensitivity and care in designing services.

Chapter 22

Assessing quality: the visit

What is required before the visit?

The framework has been designed to specify clearly what the practice is expected to produce and how it will be produced. Most criteria require a summative endpoint. It will be clear from the data whether the practice has achieved this or not. The nature of the exclusions and the reasons for omitting individual patients from lists are clear and can be a discussion point on the visit.

Summative endpoints mean that the same standards will be required and assessed across the whole country without local variation. The criteria have been selected for data that are important and should be collected anyway and therefore running an audit programme and the production of data should be a relatively small additional task for the practice. It is important that the practice knows how it is performing so that it can correct any deficiencies and does not get any surprises at the time of the visit.

Data collection for the clinical criteria

- Most by computer printout
- Practice uses same data collection tool as visitors
- No or minimum of surprises

The organisational domain requires the production of policies and some statements to prove actions have been done. The policies will be in a procedure book. The list is given in Tool 14.1. This should be available in the practice or requested beforehand to allow time for reading. Where an action or agreement with someone else is required, as in the patient survey, the practice would need to discuss the results of the questionnaire and present the agreed plan of action.

The practice is also required to demonstrate that it complies with the contractual and statutory requirements.

What is required on the day?

The practice should expect to make time available to speak to the assessors. A half-day visit is expected. This may require closure for half a day to make staff

Table 22.1 Where the assessors will look for review data.

	Look on the day	Review of presence of policy on the day	Prepared data
Clinical standards			Most by computer search and data output
Organisational standards (records)	Notes entries are made and legible. Medicines listing in record. Indication present for drugs prescribed. Reports filed in date order. Clinical summaries (*requires clinician*)	Out-of-hours data inputting Message recording Incoming communications Death notification Place for drug allergies Recording of drugs prescribed by others Policy about terminal patients' information	Smoking status and population BP recording Summaries made for new patients' notes
Organisational standards (information)	Out-of-hours telephone message	Telephone communication with professionals Stop smoking strategy Antenatal information provision	Reasons given for removal Opening hours
Organisational standards (education)	Annual appraisals occur for specified staff	Induction training Personal learning plans present for specified staff	Basic life support training Significant event reviews Annual review of complaints
Organisational standards (management)		Presence of child health surveillance policy. Computer back-up arrangements. Hepatitis B status of staff. Instrument sterilisation. Policy for advertised job specifications. Equipment maintenance. Fraud prevention. Identification of carers. Employment policies	Appointment times
Organisational standards (medicines)	Availability of prescribing history Presence of emergency drugs	Prescription availability time Follow-up of neuroleptic medication	Record of meeting prescribing advisor Prescribing review noted
Patient experience			Written report of appointment length and patient survey result and action
Additional services		Cervical smear systems and policies Child surveillance Antenatal care Emergency contraception and preconception advice	Audits of smear takers

and partners available. The assessment team from the PCO will include clinicians and managers. The PCO will have to decide who they wish to have as their visitors. The necessity to look at clinical records will require the presence of a clinician for some tasks. If the PCO simply wishes to use the visit as an assessment exercise then local managers could be used. It is likely that those organisational and patient experience criteria that require discussion with the PCO will have been achieved and signed off before the visit.

The visitors will have already viewed the written material. They may ask questions about inconsistencies in the data or the reasons for exclusion. It will be necessary to consider the expected prevalence of diseases and the prevalence reported in practice disease indexes.

Practice policies will have been seen and the visitors may discuss those policies with the practice. If there are inadequacies they can be discussed. What must be in the policies is defined by the guidance and the visitors will be aware of the detail.

Some criteria, like the legibility of the notes or the quality of summaries, will require review on the day. The detail will be specified by the contract itself and might change over time. Speaking to staff to see if they are enacted in the manner described will be a further check for some policies. This will provide triangulation that the documentation fairly represents the practice.

Tasks for the visitors

- Reviewing preparatory documentation
- Checking presence of policies
- Speaking to staff
- Review of records on the day (*requires clinician*)
- Review of other organisational standards on the day

The visitors will also require to see the practice professional development plan and understand how staff are managed and how work is devolved to staff.

Other tasks discussed on the day of the visit

The visit also provides the opportunity to discuss progress in multiple clinical areas and how the practice plans to improve in the future. It provides an opportunity to discuss with managers the resources that will be required and the other education or staff needs of the practice. This will form the basis of next year's business plan and the improvement in quality.

The PCO is responsible for IT and premises development. These are likely to be important factors in practice planning. The practice may wish to discuss how changes necessary to improve quality will affect its IT and premises requirements.

The visit provides an opportunity to discuss performance, current skills and attitudes and the future. This will be both clinical and managerial. Discussion and appraisal of managerial performance do not occur elsewhere and provide a learning opportunity. The presence of a senior manager with the ability to make decisions would greatly facilitate this process. Many practices will have improved and achieved high standards. The visit provides an opportunity to congratulate practices on a difficult task done well.

Managers also have an overview of the local NHS that practices do not have. Managers have different but complementary responsibilities for healthcare locally. In order to deliver good clinical care, practices need to become more managerial. Local NHS managers have these skills and are trying to prove achievement of the same criteria through different performance review systems. GPs can learn managerial skills and managers will benefit from understanding the clinical issues involved in improving care. The opportunity to meet and exchange information should be seen as positive.

Chapter 23

Other services bought from the practice

The practice is required to deliver essential services. It is expected to provide additional services and there are arrangements to opt in or out of these services. The criteria and standards for additional services have been defined and apply to those practices that agree to provide them in the same way as the rest of the frameworks.

Enhanced services are contracted locally although there are national contracts in some common tasks (directed and national enhanced services). They provide an opportunity for the PCO to contract for specific services from primary care. This can be for practice patients or a wider locality. Separate contracts for each one will be required which specify volume, quality criteria, personnel and training. They could be outreach services from secondary care provided in the community. The opportunity exists to provide the service using the skills and values of general practice to provide a completely different service.

This overlaps with the creation of GPwSI. This grade will provide a resource to form the backbone of the service and help with planning. GPwSI provides a route for the PCO to buy time from an individual, some of which can be used to help with planning a service, unlike the existing situation where GPs have to be paid locum fees and have difficulty releasing time. Many areas of medicine could be provided as additional services, delivering specific parts of the service that are complex and time consuming for common illnesses. Alternatively they could provide the majority of a service for diseases that are less common in which the detail of up-to-date care is not known to every GP. The training and competences of the GPwSI will be defined outside the contract.

Each service will require a contract. For those in directed and national enhanced services, these are provided. For local enhanced services, they have to be created. The principles of the GP contract are an appropriate place to start to plan those contracts. Some areas, like palliative care and mental health, are difficult to measure using summative tools and formative tools may be more appropriate.

Franchising parts of a practice

Some areas of practice would be amenable to splitting off. If resources, particularly doctor numbers, are limited it may not be possible to staff core and additional services, let alone enhanced services. In this instance patients would need to be efficiently identified as having the illnesses by the practice and care provided for those illnesses (or services; pregnancy, for instance, is not an illness) on contract elsewhere. This already happens now where some practices diagnose and refer illnesses like diabetes to secondary care for full treatment. Currently the practice would hold the full record and the primary prescribing responsibility but the latter would have to change if the service were being provided by others.

It remains to be seen whether providing care in this way can be achieved. The practice needs to provide high-quality records and registers and treat all undiagnosed illness yet would not prescribe or hold the primary record for specific illnesses. Co-ordination of prescribing for patients with multiple illnesses would become very difficult, as the only possible common record holder would not be able to decide between the different specialists.

It would be easier to manage some illnesses that rarely overlap and whose medicines don't interact. GPs or specialists could deliver this service. Patient explanations and regular follow-up of specific diseases may be possible. It would demand a radically different approach from specialists to understand the day-to-day patient issues and interactions that dominate the successful care of chronic diseases.

Working with secondary care clinicians

One of the advantages demonstrated by health maintenance organisations is the ability to introduce specialists into the community and manage a greater part of patients' care there, so reducing length of hospital stay. It is possible to manage many diseases in the community but GPs do not feel able to perform traditional hospital tasks because of the increased workload. This leads to the creation of outreach teams in the community.

They may not feel integrated into GP surgeries unless they give up their links with the hospitals. The senior members of most hospital teams are not based in the community. Consequently the resources and the sickest patients are concentrated where the senior clinicians are based – in hospital. Many patients require the facilities of the hospitals when they are ill but there is the opportunity to use enhanced services to create teams contracted directly with clinicians or their organisations to deliver specific packages of care.

The option exists of encouraging the creation of groups of secondary care doctors (and other professionals) who form a partnership ('chambers') to deliver against contracts let by the PCO for the purpose. In time these chambers would become analogous to GP practices. They could own some property and equipment but the capital costs of secondary care facilities suggest that they should use NHS facilities managed by NHS trusts for the inpatient element.

The PCO could contract directly with the 'chambers' in an analogous way to contracting with GP practices. They would function as a medical unit with consultants and partners and managers working for them. It would be possible to set quality standards in exactly the same way as the GP contract, with clinical indicators governing the payments in addition to a baseline sum.

Creating and retaining a workforce in general practice

No one knows the final configuration of the workforce. Where tasks can be delegated, they should be but the continuity of care desired by patients and the ability to consult them may produce different proportions of doctors and support staff. Work in East Kent suggests that chronic disease management is possible to this level with the existing number of GPs but there is not enough time to do the original job as well. The cost of providing services by GPs and nurses is similar. Patients should decide who provides the service.

The creation of GPwSI is assumed to take staff from general practice. However, a properly rewarded and reinvigorated general practice may retain the will of doctors to perform the generalist job and whilst some will wish to have an interest, the bulk may do the original job. There would not be a transfer out of general practice but a transfer in of specialists to provide the workforce of enhanced services. The prospect arises that enhanced services would be staffed partly from general practice and partly from specialist services. The prospect is created of specialists coming out into the community and working with GPs in the same place.

Consultants could form groups and agree contracts with PCOs to provide services for specific clinical areas. Each contract would specify the quality and outcomes to be achieved, as in the GP contract. The consultants and other secondary care staff would then gain from the autonomy and ability to manage their own environment and the close working and understanding of how much can be achieved in the community will bring benefit. Some specialists may even wish to train for a well-rewarded and reinvigorated general practice. In this way a workforce to implement a primary care-led NHS with a generalist doctor workforce can be created speedily.

Creating a general practice workforce

- Manpower requirement is not known by specialty
- Delegation is encouraged and rewarded by the contract
- Patients should decide which grade of staff they wish to see in primary care
- Enhanced services allow individual secondary care clinicians to contract to supply services
- Contracts for quality with consultants will bring benefits
- Providing services will reduce the need for GPs to leave generalist service
- Some consultants may wish to become GPs in a reinvigorated profession

General practice can be a rewarding and stimulating job. It was in the past and whether it becomes so again will depend on the decisions practices take. Income matters both as a source of money and as a reflection of how the NHS values GPs and their staff. The statements of government and the rise in spending in general practice are very encouraging. Practices have the ability to control workload and outside influence has been reduced. GPs can now be positive and start the long climb back to good recruitment and retention and a positive, forward-looking profession.

Chapter 24

Where to get help

Some practices will have managed themselves and may already be achieving most of the clinical and organisational tasks. They will need to look at the specific tasks and make some changes but are likely to be able to achieve the change required. If new staff and premises expansion are required they will need to negotiate to receive the infrastructure payments and premises amounts. For other practices at base or improving level, more help will be required.

The largest repository of talent for these issues is GPs in practices. Some practices have gone through this process, reaching very high standards in some or all areas already. In the past 'what sort of doctor' visits between practices helped development. It would be entirely appropriate to encourage meetings between GPs, staff and practice managers to swap ideas and implementation methods. This is the kind of professional activity that leads to the development of values and local leaders to take change forward. Colleagues will not be able to provide large amounts of time for tutoring others unpaid and therefore detailed development work will require a sponsoring organisation. The benefits to an improving practice in financial terms are substantial and the cost of a colleague's time to facilitate this is a good investment.

Sources of help

- PCO management experience
- GP tutors
- Colleagues in practices are a useful resource
- Payment to release time is required
  - Can be achieved through PCO
  - RCGP formative schemes
  - Private consultancy

PCO

Benchmarking of the existing situation using the clinical and organisational framework as described in education and training will produce a list of tasks and competences to be accomplished. The PCO employs medical and managerial staff with experience of practice development.

Some of the criteria require implementation of local policies. PCOs could be expected to have model policies and make copies freely available to practices.

Many PCOs already pay for external facilitation of change by employing management consultants or the RCGP (through QTD). If the skills are in the area already practices could request the PCO to pay in advance for GP or staff time to spend with, or in, another practice assisting with development. This is difficult as the aim is to help the practice understand itself and develop skills. It is not to do the task for them. If practices solve their own problems then permanent improvement will occur and new skills will be developed.

The PCO also employs appraisers. This is intended to be a personal formative review of educational needs. It represents an opportunity to openly discuss educational needs and plan for the future. Such is the size of the agenda for some practices that there may also be a need to scale down expectations and plans to allow development over a longer period to reduce or prevent stress-related problems.

Regional postgraduate structure

A number of staff are employed and supported by this structure. Most relate to registrars but the skills are similar. The local GP tutor also provides an independent source of advice on where to go for education. If a common agenda emerges from practices, the GP tutor could facilitate meetings and arrange speakers.

RCGP

The RCGP already has a number of quality schemes that guide and support practice development. Each is different and has been developed from a different source. Whilst that can give difficulty with co-ordination, it also provides a rich source of different ideas and criteria derived in different ways. Each one provides a mixture of formative and summative criteria to use to benchmark performance and steer new work towards improvement. Some of the schemes provide local mentors to read initial presentations and help with preparation of material. These mentors have experience as principals in practice and of the assessment process itself. Their input can be used to improve performance and, if the advice is followed, produce work that will be likely to be approved when PCO assessors review the practice.

The college schemes are intended to be completed by individuals, leading to a personal award, or the practice, leading to practice-based accreditations. All are by peers and there is lay involvement in the assessments. Consequently GPs and lay representation are involved for all and managers are also involved in practice assessments. The person-based schemes Fellowship by Assessment (FBA) and Membership by Assessment of Performance (MAP) review a substantial number of practice attributes because good practice is impossible in a poor environment and GPs have control over that environment. They also contain peer review of personal clinical skills, most of which are formative.

The practice-based assessments QTD and QPA have criteria and standards similar to the organisational domain. Currently QTD is almost all formative and it will help development but there is no certainty of the level reached because it is formative. QPA is a mix of summative and formative. These schemes can be used in conjunction with the summative criteria to provide help in reaching the level. A summative standard can also be used as proof that a level has been reached and accepted in place of measuring the organisational standard on the day. Once a scheme had been achieved the practice would retain the skills and opt to produce data for the organisational framework because they already had the skills in house to achieve and maintain that level. The practice may wish to enrol for another assessment that was different at a later date.

The faculty structure of the college exists and their assessors are likely to be known to the faculty. Others with an interest in quality practice, education and registrars are also likely to be involved. The faculty could provide a common local point of contact to facilitate individual visits or networking of those involved with assessment and quality improvement. The networking between individuals with different assessment backgrounds will benefit all the assessment schemes.

Private consultancy

There are many other possible sources of advice for practices. Which they choose to use is up to them in the contract structure. The budget for practice development is contained within the global sum and rises as development occurs. It is therefore the practice choice whether to involve an outside agency. However, those resources specifically recognised in the contract or by the NHS – PCO advice, GP tutor input, QPA and in some PCOs QTD – will be separately funded and no or low cost options to the practice.

Chapter 25

What happens next

The act of publishing the Quality and Outcomes Framework raised the profile of specific clinical, organisational and patient-related issues. GPs and managers audited their own performance in order to decide whether to vote for the contract.

The majority of primary care education and development will relate to the contract agenda. New people and systems will come into place to help the practices in the most difficult areas with the most development to achieve. In time change will occur for all, some at a very rapid pace and others slower, but substantial improvement will be delivered over time.

In the process of achieving the criteria in the framework, new structures and skills will be developed in primary care. These skills are generic and can and will be used to develop new services. The stability of the income will allow individuals and practices to look at new developments. Some will work, some will not. This experience will be used as the basis for further development.

Will chronic disease management take over general practice?

Surveys of the public show that they continue to trust doctors and GPs in particular. Patients feel they have their 'own GP' and GPs refer to their 'own patients'. It is essentially a personal relationship that lasts many years and there is a high satisfaction rating with practices. Patients have a trust in the organisation of general practice (public trust) and a trust in the individual (personal trust). Both will need to be retained if patients are to co-operate with practices to improve the management of illness.

The contract will change the focus of practices. There are worries about a move away from personal care and into chronic disease management alone. However, two of the drivers of change, improving patient care and professional pride, are related to personal care and the personal relationship between a GP and their patient.

In time the values of continuity and trust will reassert themselves at a new and higher level of chronic disease management because the longitudinal relationship is beneficial to both parties. It is questionable whether patients would repeatedly attend for structured disease care unless they had confidence in the individuals delivering the care.

Personal observation suggests that similar relationships exist with practice nurses, district nurses, health visitors and other primary care staff. Ultimately success with chronic disease management means using the personal trust patients have in their doctor or practice staff to achieve a difficult change. That personal trust will need to be refreshed after the contract is achieved by the public seeing the improvement in public health and a re-establishment of the personal doctor–patient trust built through continuity and care for the patient as an individual. Whilst the contract with the NHS is to be with the practice, patients are likely to continue to feel that they have a personal contract with GPs and primary care staff.

Who manages the practice?

The contract is between the PCO and the practice. The practice needs to employ a GP but there is no necessity for the contract to be exclusively between GP partners and the PCO. The requirements to be a partner and manage the practice are considerable. Some GPs wish to do this as it is the act of managing that gives autonomy and the ability to produce patient-focused healthcare. Some may not or the demands may be too great. It will be costly for GPs to take time out of practice to attend meetings and be involved in strategic management.

In time partners may delegate more and more work to managers who will need to be brought into the business as partners. They would then be asked to participate in providing the capital of the business. There is nothing to stop the practice becoming a limited company and working across multiple surgeries. It would need to consider how to get the best from its workforce and how to involve clinicians.

Alternatively other clinicians in primary care could take on partnership responsibilities. Nurses, pharmacists and other clinicians may wish to help run the business.

Using the opportunities to improve quality of life

The reason why the profession requested a new contract was the low morale and high workload of practices. The contract also seeks to deliver a rise in incomes for primary care staff and an increase in resources and capability. Devolving responsibility to practices allows them to organise themselves and make choices about income and workload.

The development agenda will see a major improvement in the management ability in practices. Creating an organisation capable of achieving high levels on the Quality and Outcomes Framework is something GP and PCO managers should take pride in.

The managers of the practices, GP partners and employees have an opportunity to improve their own working lives and those around them. It will not be easy but there is a substantial prize on offer. When practices achieve this, recruitment and retention will improve and a 'virtuous' cycle can start again with practices proud of their good recruitment record and growing numbers of GPs, managers and nurses.

Reviewing and updating the contract

The contract will require some review. Some of the wording of criteria may need adjusting in the light of experience or gradual improvement in the evidence may suggest a change to the detail of some criteria. New legislation may render some criteria inadequate or redundant. These gradual changes could produce significant alterations over time. All existing quality schemes are upgraded in this way.

Alternatively there could be the sudden development of a safety problem with a whole class of drugs. If this were ACE inhibitors or statins then the existing Medicines Control Agency safety arrangements would be used. Several contract criteria would be instantly rendered impossible and the framework would need to be altered to reflect this.

The old contract became out of date because nearly all practices had achieved the quality measures of the time (smears, maternity care, etc.) and the contract ceased to discriminate between practices on the quality of service provided. When most practices are achieving the criteria to steady-state levels, then the new contract will require an overhaul. Such is the challenge and difficulty of the contract that this is likely to be some way into the future.

Reasons to review the contract

- Need to increase clarity
- Emergence of severe side effects with particular groups of drugs or treatments
- Changes in legislation or regulation
- Changes to the evidence base
- Change in the level of criteria as they become less sensitive as indicators between practices

---

Constraints on new criteria

There is not a great deal more usable clinical evidence to create additional summative criteria. In time the process of creating evidence in medicine could change. It is to be hoped that evidence will be trialled in normal populations before being promulgated for general introduction. This would be a significant and beneficial change in the use of evidence in medicine.

The patient experience does not need to change because it consists of consultation with patients. In time the views of patients will change but the structure does not need to. Similarly, the wording of the contractual and statutory requirements will not change but the tasks described will evolve.

The organisational domain could be changed or expanded. The current framework consists of broadly developmental indicators. Success with the standards develops the practice. It could also be changed from a developmental framework by adding criteria that force specific tasks on practice, for example if a large number of criteria were introduced forcing attendance at specific meetings or the presence of a piece of equipment. A list of tasks that seemed important at the time in their own right would be created. This would produce difficulties if the autonomy of method were taken away. It would be worse if GPs felt the tasks did not help patient care. Cutting across the five drivers would damage the framework.

Conversely if the new criteria provided the five drivers and extended the contract into new areas, significant improvement could result. The option of using QPA and other formative quality schemes in this context is also important. This and the other RCGP schemes evolve because they are constantly updated. In time the areas of the contract that were not amenable to the creation of summative standards could be included as formative standards.

At some date in the future a new framework may be required when general practice achieves the standards of the contract across the whole country. It would be a matter for congratulation that such a challenging agenda had been designed, implemented and achieved.

Part 4

Tool box

Chapter 26

Tools to understand what is happening now

This book has developed a number of themes. The practice has to understand what it is currently achieving and the methods it is using for IT, staff, education planning and business planning before it can make changes.

In order to understand the current position it is helpful to start with a list of the significant factors in any given area and review the current activity of the practice.

This can be done by an individual reviewing a list privately and scoring it. Any factors the individual feels are important can be changed over time. Alternatively, a group of people could consider the list and by discussion produce consensus. There is also the possibility that the views of the group will change at the time or later.

If desired, the list could be turned into a questionnaire and given to the relevant group of staff or partners and the result tabulated, for an individual or a group. Feedback of the results to those who filled in the questionnaire, with a personal score and the scores of others, would give individuals an understanding of where their answers differ from others. Discussion of the results among the wider group may produce further understanding and possibly change. A questionnaire to determine staff and clinician confidence with the practice computer system is provided in Tool 26.1.

Ways to use the tools

- Individual consideration of personal or practice performance
- Group discussion and rating of personal and practice performance
- Creation of questionnaires
- Feedback of questionnaire results
- Group discussion of findings

Outcomes of using tools

- Personal understanding and desire to change
- Group understanding of personal and others' views
- Peer pressure to change
- Group decision to change

Tools to understand the current situation are distributed throughout the book:

- Tool 12.1 Understanding the management of a practice – *see* p. 115.
- Tool 13.1 Practice IT staff competences – *see* p. 124.
- Tool 14.1 Policies required from the practice – *see* p. 131.
- Tool 14.2 Staff functions required in the practice – *see* p. 133.
- Tool 14.3 Practice systems to encourage quality of working – *see* p. 134.
- Tool 17.1 Issues to be considered in organising a questionnaire survey – *see* p. 156.

An additional tool to list the clinical areas that the contract focuses on is provided – *see* pp. 209–11.

Tool 26.2 has two empty columns, where to find guidelines and mechanism to harmonise practice. These will vary over time as medicine develops and guidelines change. Initially it will be possible to use the supporting guidance for the contract to find guidelines, in time it will be necessary to look in a number of authoritative sources. Similarly because practices vary there is no single method for each clinical area that will guarantee to update practitioners. It is expected that practices will create their own solutions. The table can be used as a template to fill in the source of guidelines to be used and the method of communicating best practice to members of the practice.

Tools in Chapters 26 and 27 are available at www.radcliffe-oxford.com/qualitygms in a format that can be used as working documents to implement change.

Tool 26.1   Questionnaire on use of computers in clinical situations

In order to assess how the practice might improve the use of IT in clinical situations, it is necessary to understand the abilities within the practice. We can only do so if we all have training appropriate to our needs. As a first step I would like to gather information about how we use the system now. *Please be as accurate as possible.* (This is not a competition!)

1   Which of the following best describes your own attitude to using the computer when consulting patients?

- Prefer not to use it at all
- Use it to print scripts
- Access some information but mostly refer to paper records
- Find the information useful but don't often add much detail to it
- Find information useful and usually add data when recorded
- Regular use of data and detailed recording of all appropriate data necessary for clinical management
- Regular use of data and detailed recording to the extent that no paper record could ever be considered necessary (remembering possible queries should complaints, etc. arise)

2   Which best describes your ability to record appropriate information during consultations?

- Not confident recording any data
- Confident to some extent in recording the following (please indicate on a scale of 1–10 your confidence, speed and willingness to add each of the items listed: 1 = a struggle but might just achieve it, 10 = slick operation)

	1	2	3	4	5	6	7	8	9	10
Computer printing an acute or repeat prescription										
Adding a BP										
Read coding other symptoms/signs										
Read coding a diagnosis										
Finding and reviewing a blood test or X-ray										
Using a template to enter data										
Adding a clinical comment on a consultation										
Adding to a disease register										
Checking and amending a summary or problem list										
Adding health promotion information										
Altering a repeat medication										
Adding an indication for a medication										
Recording a medication review										
Recording a chronic disease review										
Printing information leaflets for patients										
Finding referral and hospital letters on computer										
Using Internet access for information during consultations										

3 What factors limit the extent to which you record information?

4 Are there data you would like to access on the system which you are unskilled in locating?

5 If so, what data?

6 What aspects of IT give you most problems?

7 How keen are you to add to your data-handling skills?

8 What other IT skills do you need?
   - Word processing
   - Using the clinical resources in the practice computer
   - Accessing libraries and journals on the Internet
   - Email
   - Other

Tool 26.2 Education and training requirement for the clinical criteria

Possible education requirement	Medical knowledge required	Treatments, contraindications, interactions and monitoring	Ability to explain the reasons for treatment to patients Materials Lifestyle	Where to find authoritative guidelines to adapt for local use	Meeting or mechanism to swap knowledge and harmonise practice
Disease area					
Angina	Disease and prognosis Exercise testing Control of cholesterol Antiplatelet drugs Control of BP Influenza vaccination	Statins and other lipid-lowering treatments Aspirin and other antiplatelet drugs Beta-blockers	Disease and prognosis Diagnostic tests Smoking cessation		
MI	Disease and prognosis Control of cholesterol Antiplatelet drugs Control of BP Influenza vaccination	Statins and other lipid-lowering treatments Aspirin and other antiplatelet drugs Beta-blockers ACE inhibitors	Disease and prognosis Diagnostic tests Smoking cessation		
Left ventricular dysfunction	Disease and prognosis Diagnostic methods and differential diagnosis	ACE inhibitors	Disease and prognosis Diagnostic tests		
Stroke and TIA	Disease and prognosis Diagnostic methods Control of cholesterol Antiplatelet drugs Control of BP Influenza vaccination	Statins and other lipid-lowering treatments Aspirin and other antiplatelet drugs	Disease and prognosis Diagnostic tests Smoking cessation		

Tool 26.2 Continued.

Possible education requirement	Medical knowledge required	Treatments, contraindications, interactions and monitoring	Ability to explain the reasons for treatment to patients Materials Lifestyle	Where to find authoritative guidelines to adapt for local use	Meeting or mechanism to swap knowledge and harmonise practice
Hypertension	Disease and prognosis Diagnostic methods	Major groups of drugs used and detailed knowledge for the commonly used drugs to enable confidence in co-prescribing	Disease and prognosis Diagnostic criteria		
Diabetes mellitus	Disease and prognosis Diagnostic methods Control of HbA1c Control of weight Control of cholesterol Control of BP Retinal problems Peripheral pulses Neuropathy testing Renal function testing Micro-albuminuria testing Influenza vaccination	Antidiabetic treatments Statins and other lipid-lowering treatments Aspirin and other antiplatelet drugs Beta-blockers ACE inhibitors	Disease and prognosis Diagnostic criteria Smoking cessation Weight control Diet control		
COPD	Disease and prognosis Diagnostic methods Spirometry Influenza vaccination		Disease and prognosis Diagnostic criteria Smoking cessation Inhaler technique		

Condition		
Epilepsy	Disease and prognosis Diagnostic methods Reasons for medication review	Disease and prognosis Reasons for being fit free
Hypothyroidism	Disease and prognosis Reasons for reviewing thyroid function tests (TFT) When to change treatment based on TFT	Disease and prognosis Reasons for reviewing TFT Support needs
Cancer	Diseases and prognosis Diagnostic methods What should be in a review Co-ordination arrangements with secondary care	
Severe long-term mental health problems	Diseases and prognosis Diagnostic methods What should be in a review	Support needs Physical health review
Lithium therapy	Lithium therapy Reason for TSH and creatinine review	
Asthma	Diseases and prognosis Diagnostic methods What should be in a review Influenza vaccination	Disease and prognosis Diagnostic criteria Smoking cessation Inhaler technique

Chapter 27

Tools to help change

Once an individual, a group within the practice or the whole practice decides it understands what is happening now and wants to change, it has to have a method. In order to do this it needs to decide on relevant areas and methods. The criteria of the contract are a good place to start to assess what needs to change. It is not an exclusive list and there are many important areas not covered. Other areas of importance or criteria can be added or subtracted from the list as desired.

For each criterion the practice needs to decide if it is already satisfactorily achieving it. If it is not but wishes to then someone needs to be given the task of producing change. In addition there needs to be a mechanism in the practice management team for reviewing progress and a person who takes strategic responsibility for the task. The management team may comprise different groups of people in different practices but will usually include the practice manager and partners. It may also include a manager outside the practice or a junior manager within the practice, depending on practice size.

Once responsibility is determined then a method of achieving the change needs to be put in place. This will include changes in the structure of the practice (buildings, equipment and staff) as well as function (ways of working policies and internal protocols). There is also likely to be a training requirement arising from the consideration of each criterion. This can be divided up and allocated as training for individuals.

The list of training requirements for the whole practice can be used to create the practice professional development plan whilst the individual training plans are personal development plans. The expected changes to structure, function and education become the practice business plan. As the various plans are created by rewriting the objectives produced by this process, priorities can be decided and a timescale given to the plan. Business planning will require checking that the changes to structure and function are occurring in a planned way with the relevant staff and infrastructure in place at the correct time to be used.

Tools are provided to:

- Assess performance for the criteria in the contract either individually or in groups
- Allocate responsibility
- Describe structural change required
- Describe functional change required
- Describe education required
- Relate functional and structural change over time
- Produce a practice education plan
- Produce personal development plans.

Some are in this tool box section and some are referenced back to methods and tables in the text. This gives the ability to plan the required change using the criteria but it is not a list of protocols or management strategies to achieve the change itself.

Tools to assist business planning
See text of Chapter 19 for suggested methods.

Tools to create new criteria
See Chapter 6 on creating indicators and standards.

Tools to prepare for the visit
Tool 14.1   Policies required from the practice – *see* p. 131.
Table 22.1 Where the assessors will look for review data – *see* p. 188.

Tool 27.1   Planning to achieve clinical criteria

Organisational standard	Is it happening already?	Who should do this task?	Responsible person?	Structural change required?	Skills required?	Training or course required?
IT						
Cleaning the disease registers						
Adding to the disease registers						
Entering data to the computer already recorded in the paper records						
Seeing the patients requiring care						
Number and nature of disease management clinics						
Writing practice policies						
Writing patient group directions						
Number of additional doctors required						
Number of additional nurses required						
Number of additional team members, e.g. pharmacist						
Infrastructure implications						
Number of computer terminals						
Capacity of central server, IT system provider						
Nature of computer peripherals, back-up method, printers, other software available						
Number of receptionists required						
Demand for prescriptions						
Management support for the larger practice						
Staff						
Changes are present in organisational criteria						

Tool 27.2 Planning to achieve organisational criteria

Contractual and statutory requirements	Is it happening already?	Who should do this task?	Responsible person?	Structural change required?	Skills required?	Training or course required?
Organisational standard The practice has an agreed procedure for handling patients' complaints which complies with the NHS complaints procedure and is advertised to the patients.						
Where patients are requesting to join the practice list, the practice does not discriminate on the grounds of: 1 race, gender, social class, age, religion, sexual orientation or appearance 2 disability or medical condition.						
The practice adheres to the requirements of the Medicines Act for the storage, prescribing, dispensing, recording and disposal of drugs, including controlled drugs.						
Batch numbers are recorded for all vaccines administered.						
The practice has a policy for consent to the treatment of children that conforms to the current Children Act or equivalent legislation.						
The premises, equipment and arrangements for infection control and decontamination meet the minimum national standards.						
The practice ensures that all healthcare professionals who are employed by the practice are currently registered with the relevant professional body on the appropriate part(s) of its Register(s) and that any employed general practitioner is a member of a recognised medical defence organisation and registered on a primary care performers list (or equivalent).						

All professionals working in the practice are covered by appropriate indemnity insurance.

All doctors have an annual appraisal.

The practice has a system to allow patients access to their records on request in accordance with current legislation.

There is a designated individual (data controller) responsible for confidentiality.

If the records are computerised there are mechanisms to ensure that the data are transferred when patients leave the practice.

If the team uses a computer, it is registered under and conforms to the provisions of the Data Protection Act.

The practice has a written procedure for the electronic transmission of patient data which is in line with national policy.

The practice complies with current legislation on employment rights and discrimination.

All staff have written terms and conditions of employment conforming to or exceeding the statutory minimum.

The practice meets the statutory requirements of the Health & Safety at Work Act and complies with the current Approved Code of Practice in Management of Health and Safety at Work Regulations.

Vaccines are stored in accordance with manufacturers' instructions.

Individual healthcare professionals should be able to demonstrate that they comply with the national child protection guidance, and should provide at least one critical event analysis regarding concerns about a child's welfare if appropriate.

Tool 27.2   Continued.

Contractual and statutory requirements	Is it happening already?	Who should do this task?	Responsible person?	Structural change required?	Skills required?	Training or course required?
All practices have in place systems of clinical governance which enable quality assurance of their services and promote quality improvement and enhanced patient safety.						
The underpinning structures within the practice should ensure embedding of clinical governance through a nominated clinical governance lead.						
For minor surgery, patients' consent to any surgical procedures, including wart cautery and joint injections, is recorded.						
For vaccination and immunisation, consent to immunisation, or contraindications if they exist, are recorded in the records.						
For vaccination and immunisation, fridges in which vaccines are stored have a maximum thermometer daily reading on working days.						
For vaccination and immunisation, staff involved in administering vaccines are trained in the recognition of anaphylaxis and able to administer appropriate first-line treatment when it occurs.						

Tool 27.3 Planning to achieve patient experience criteria

Organisational standard	Is it happening already?	Who should do this task?	Responsible person?	Structural change required?	Skills required?	Training or course required?
Records and information about patients						
Each patient contact with a clinician is recorded in the patient's record, including consultations, visits and telephone advice.						
Entries in the records are legible.						
The practice has a system for transferring and acting on information about patients seen by other doctors out of hours.						
There is a reliable system to ensure that messages and requests for visits are recorded and that the appropriate doctor or team member receives and acts upon them.						
The practice has a system for dealing with any hospital report or investigation results which identifies a responsible health professional and ensures that any necessary action is taken.						
There is a system for ensuring that the relevant team members are informed about patients who have died.						
The medicines that a patient is receiving are clearly listed in their record.						
There is a designated place for the recording of drug allergies and adverse reactions in the notes and these are clearly recorded.						
For repeat medicines, an indication for the drug can be identified in the records (for drugs added to repeat prescription with effect from 1 April 2004).						

Tool 27.3   Continued.

Organisational standard	Is it happening already?	Who should do this task?	Responsible person?	Structural change required?	Skills required?	Training or course required?
The smoking status of patients aged 15–75 is recorded.						
The blood pressure of patients aged 45 and over is recorded in the preceding five years.						
When a member of the team prescribes a medicine other than a non-medicated dressing, topical treatment or over-the-counter (OTC) medicine, there is a mechanism for that prescription to be entered into the patient's general practice record.						
There is a system to alert the out-of-hours service or duty doctor to patients dying at home.						
The records, hospital letters and investigation reports are filed in date order or available electronically in date order.						
The practice has up-to-date clinical summaries.						
Newly registered patients have had their notes summarised within eight weeks of receipt by the practice.						
Patient communication						
The practice has a system to allow patients to contact the out-of-hours service by making no more than two telephone calls.						
If an answering system is used out of hours, the message is clear and the contact number is given at least twice.						

The practice has arrangements for patients to speak to GPs and nurses on the telephone during the working day.

If a patient is removed from a practice's list, the practice provides an explanation of the reasons in writing to the patient and information on how to find a new practice, unless it is perceived such an action would result in a violent response by the patient.

The practice supports smokers in stopping by a strategy, which includes providing literature and offering appropriate therapy.

Information is available to patients on the roles of the GP, community midwife, health visitor and hospital clinics in the provision of antenatal and postnatal care.

Patients are able to access a receptionist via telephone and face to face in the practice, for at least 45 hours over five days, Monday to Friday, except where agreed with the PCO.

The practice has a system to allow patients to contact the out-of-hours service by making no more than one telephone call.

Education and training

There is a record of all practice-employed clinical staff having attended training/updating in basic life support skills in the preceding 18 months.

Practice-employed nurses have an annual appraisal.

New staff receive induction training.

There is a record of all practice-employed staff having attended training/updating in basic life support skills in the preceding 36 months.

Tool 27.3 Continued.

Organisational standard	Is it happening already?	Who should do this task?	Responsible person?	Structural change required?	Skills required?	Training or course required?
The practice conducts an annual review of patient complaints and suggestions to ascertain general learning points which are shared with the team.						
The practice has undertaken a minimum of 12 significant event reviews in the past three years which include (if these have occurred): • Any death occurring in the practice premises • Two new cancer diagnoses • Two deaths where terminal care has taken place at home • One patient complaint • One suicide • One section under the Mental Health Act.						
All practice-employed nurses have personal learning plans which have been reviewed at annual appraisal.						
All practice-employed non-clinical team members have an annual appraisal.						
Practice management Individual healthcare professionals have access to information on local procedures relating to child protection.						
There are clearly defined arrangements for backing up computer data, back-up verification, safe storage of back-up tapes and authorisation for loading programs where a computer is used.						

The hepatitis B status of all doctors and relevant practice-employed staff is recorded and immunisation recommended if required in accordance with national guidance.

The arrangements for instrument sterilisation comply with national guidelines as applicable to primary care.

The practice offers a range of appointment times to patients which, as a minimum, should include morning and afternoon appointments five mornings and four afternoons per week except where agreed with the PCO.

Person specifications and job descriptions are produced for all advertised vacancies.

The practice has systems in place to ensure regular and appropriate inspection, calibration, maintenance and replacement of equipment including:

- a defined responsible person
- clear recording
- systematic pre-planned schedules
- reporting of faults.

The practice has a policy to ensure the prevention of fraud and has defined levels of financial responsibility and accountability for staff undertaking financial transactions (accounts, payroll, drawings, payment of invoices, signing cheques, petty cash, pensions, superannuation, etc.).

The practice has a protocol for the identification of carers and a mechanism for the referral of carers for social services assessment.

There is a written procedure manual that includes staff employment policies, including equal opportunities, bullying and harassment and sickness absence (including illegal drugs, alcohol and stress) to which staff have access.

Tool 27.3 Continued.

Organisational standard	Is it happening already?	Who should do this task?	Responsible person?	Structural change required?	Skills required?	Training or course required?
Medicines management						
Details of prescribed medicines are available to the prescriber at each surgery consultation.						
The practice possesses the equipment and up-to-date emergency drugs to treat anaphylaxis.						
There is a system for checking expiry dates of emergency drugs at least on an annual basis.						
The number of hours from requesting a prescription to availability for collection by the patient is known.						
Where the practice has responsibility for administering regular injectable neuroleptic medication, there is a system to identify and follow up patients who do not attend.						
A medication review is recorded in the notes in the preceding 15 months for all patients being prescribed repeat medicines (excluding OTC and topical medications).						
The practice meets with the PCO prescribing advisor at least annually, has agreed up to three actions related to prescribing and subsequently provided evidence of change.						
Additional services						
1 Cervical screening						
The percentage of patients aged 25–64 years (in Scotland 25–60 years) whose notes record that a cervical smear has been performed in the last 3–5 years.						
The practice has a system to ensure inadequate/abnormal smears are followed up.						

The practice has a policy on how to identify and follow up cervical smear defaulters and can record when patients wish to be excluded from cervical smears.

Women who have opted for exclusion from the cervical cytology recall register must be offered the opportunity to change their decision at least every five years.

The practice has a system for informing all women of the results of cervical smears.

The practice has a policy for auditing its cervical screening service, and performs an audit of inadequate cervical smears in relation to individual smear takers at least every two years.

2 Child health surveillance

Child development checks are offered at the intervals agreed in local guidelines and problems are followed up.

3 Maternity services

Antenatal care and screening are offered according to current local guidelines.

4 Contraceptive services

The team has a written policy for responding to requests for emergency contraception.

The team has a policy for providing pre-conceptual advice.

Patient experience

Patient questionnaire.

Reflecting on the patient questionnaire and making changes.

Consulting with patients or PCO.

Setting up patient participation group.

Ten-minute appointments.

Tool 27.4 Planning to achieve criteria common to several domains

Organisational requirement	Is it happening already?	Who should do this task?	Responsible person?	Structural change required?	Skills required?	Training or course required?
Common requirements across all domains						
Education requirement						
Creating a practice professional development plan						
Requirement for education meetings					–	–
Business planning						
Creating a business plan						
Requirement for planning meetings					–	–

Further information

For the clinical criteria there are a number of sources of information. The major ones are listed but the supporting documentation for the contract[41] lists references for each clinical criteria and sources of information.

The **National electronic Library for Health** brings together journals and libraries and has an extensive range of guidelines.
www.nelh.nhs.uk/

The **National Institute for Clinical Excellence** creates the authoritative guidance for England and Wales.
www.nice.nhs.uk/

The **Scottish Intercollegiate Guideline Network** creates the authoritative guidance for Scotland.
www.sign.ac.uk

The **Royal College of General Practitioners** site has details of its quality schemes.
www.rcgp.org

The **Institute of Healthcare Management** site has contact details for its quality scheme.
www.ihm.org.uk

The **Health Quality Service** site has details of its primary care quality scheme.
www.hqs.org.uk

The **National Association for Patient Participation** site has details and instructions on how to set up a patient participation group.
www.napp.org.uk

The **Business Link** (a government agency for the business community) site has details of current employment law and staff policies as well as ideas about business planning.
www.businesslink.org

The **ACAS** site has details and advice about employment issues.
www.acas.org.uk

Index